GNVQ Advanced Options

Human Behaviour in the Caring Context

Neil Moonie • Graham Ixer

Kate Makepeace • Indira Balkissoon

Havering College of Further and Higher Education, Essex

Published in 1995 by
Stanley Thornes (Publishers) Ltd
Ellenborough House
Wellington Street
Cheltenham
Glos. GL50 1YD
United Kingdom

A catalogue record for this book is available from The British Library.

ISBN 0 7487 1769 2

Typeset by GCS, Leighton Buzzard
Printed and bound in Great Britain by Scotprint, Musselburgh

Contents

Acknowledgements

The authors and publishers are grateful to the following for permission to reproduce material:
Hulton Deutsch Collection Limited, page 155; John Birdsall Photography, pages 22, 66, 120, 161, 174; Mirror Syndication International, page 156; Penguin Books Ltd, page 78; Pictor International Ltd, cover photo; Popperfoto, page 63.

Introduction

This book has been written to support students studying for the GNVQ Advanced qualification in Health and Social Care. Specifically the book is designed to support the BTEC Optional Units 10 and 13, and RSA Unit 15. The first four chapters are designed to support study of BTEC Unit 10, 'Human Behaviour in the Context of Health and Social Care'. Chapters 5, 6 and 7 are designed to support BTEC Unit 13, 'Investigate Work Groups in Care Organisations'. Besides supporting the optional units, this text may also contribute to BTEC additional unit study. Because this text focuses on two units, a Section Summary and References are provided at the conclusion of each unit section.

This book is not designed as a manual of information for candidates to reference. There are several existing works in the field of psychology and group work which provide good general reference material for academic study. This book is designed with quite a different purpose in mind.

We believe that GNVQ provides an opportunity to review the use of academic knowledge in relation to vocational issues. Health and Social Care represents a valid focus for academic learning in its own right. Research and knowledge gained in the context of academic disciplines now need to be related to the vocation of Health and Social Care. Received knowledge should be evaluated for its usefulness and relevance to Health and Social Care practice.

The book represents quite an ambitious project in that it seeks to break new ground, not in terms of its content, but in terms of its perspective. GNVQs are neither traditional discipline based qualifications, nor are they aimed at achieving competence. GNVQ qualifications are based on standards of achievement. This new approach to vocational learning provides an opportunity to explore the use of concepts in Health and Social Care. This book explores concepts which may underpin an advanced level understanding of human behaviour in the social care context.

In trying to achieve its purpose the book has not followed the organisation of the standards. Standards are designed for assessment purposes, not as a guide for learning. Some aspects of standards are not covered in the book; for example, research techniques, as these are very well covered by texts for the mandatory units. On the other hand, this text deliberately introduces material which is not to be found in the optional standards. The book centres on an initial description of the NVQ value base. Our reasoning is that this value base provides a focus for evaluating the use of concepts in caring; the value base is integrated into the Mandatory Units, but it seemed more appropriate to reference the vocational value base directly.

This book is focused on BTEC optional unit standards and so the authors have mainly attempted to cover those issues required by the standards. The authors are also aware that some users will be looking for a quick explanation of theories and concepts; rather than an evaluation of their application. To this end we have constructed 'Section Summary' sections to provide coverage of the terminology employed in the 1994 optional standards.

In summary, this book is designed to explore human behaviour in the caring context;

we hope it will also answer a need for quick reference. We have not written another textbook on psychology or group work, nor have we constructed some kind of definitive manual of Health and Social Care theory.

SECTION ONE

1 Using theories of self in caring

What is covered in this chapter

- The quality of care and the concept of empowerment
- The NVQ value base
- Understanding self-concept and identity
- Social influences on self
- Imagining a 'me'
- The concept of social role
- Self-actualisation
- Using theories
- Theories of self – an evaluation
- Identity and empowerment

The quality of care and the concept of empowerment

Reflective activity

Imagine that you go on holiday to a far distant country, you become ill, perhaps you have been unconscious. You are taken into hospital for checks but you don't know what is wrong with you. You are alone and don't know exactly where you are or what will happen – there are no other people to talk to. In this situation, how important would the following things be? Imagine them in order of priority.

- Having good quality furniture around you.
- Having a reasonable size room.
- Being able to choose your own food from a menu.
- Having someone who was warm and friendly who would spend time talking to you and giving you information.
- Being treated with respect and consulted about what you thought was best for you in the way of treatment.

Now think about fear – if you are alone in a strange place as described – how unpleasant and frightening would the following things be? Imagine them in order of unpleasantness.

- Not being talked to – being ignored if you asked questions.
- Being criticised about the way you look physically.
- Being told it was your own fault that you were ill and that it will teach you a lesson.
- Not being given a choice of food or clothes – being told what to eat.
- Having people discuss your details and make comments but not talking to you.

Looking at the first list on p. 3, many people would be much more concerned with the quality of consultation and conversation than they would be about the size of the room. Some people would be concerned about furniture and room size because it may indicate something about the way a person is valued; or something about the quality of service. If a person is alone or afraid, conversation, choice and consultation may prove far more effective in making that person feel valued than the simple surroundings. Looking at the second list, they all seem fairly awful – different people have their own worst fears. Some people would find the direct discrimination of being criticised about appearance or blamed for needing care as most offensive.

People require care services because they have some area of vulnerability. A person requires health care services because of an illness or disability, or life event which they cannot completely cope with alone. A person will use social care services because there are areas of social need or daily living problems which require support. As in the imaginary situation above, many service users will feel vulnerable or feel at risk. Good quality caring will address this vulnerability.

Good quality care will make service users or 'clients' feel valued. National Vocational Qualifications in Caring are centred on the principle of promoting equality for all individuals. No units can be awarded without this principle being assessed as part of the practice. GNVQs include this principle both in the mandatory units and in performance criteria throughout the qualification.

Promoting equality would result in equal control, or equal power being shared between the client and the carer. The client might feel like a person who is ill in a distant country. Even so, instead of feeling at risk or feeling vulnerable to the staff who look after them, the client should feel that they are equal to the staff. The staff have power to influence the quality of life of the client. But this power could be shared with clients so that the client is 'empowered'. A central principle of good quality care is that carers should empower clients. It is important to note that not all care services are empowering. For example:

> One study of a London borough's provision of residential care for elders reported:
> - Elders being woken up between 5.45 and 6.30 in the morning without choice.
> - Lack of choice about when to go to bed.
> - Lack of opportunity to get drinks and snacks when wanted.
> - Lack of choice and consultation about meals.
> - No choice over bringing in personal possessions, no personal furniture, telephone, TV or radio.
> - No procedures for washing, mending and marking personal belongings or clothing.
> - Lack of attention to clothing which was often allowed to become dirty.
> (S. Tomlin, 1989, p. 11)

Such a service is disempowering. The residents had no choice over key events in their daily life. The lack of personal possessions and lack of attention to clothing also suggest a general lack of value for clients.

How does this actual study compare with your own fears in the first exercise?

Why is care sometimes disempowering?

There are a range of issues which can be reviewed here. On a personal level, care is sometimes given in terms of the carer's experience of care.

Most people have experienced being cared for as children. Adults often take control (and power) over children because they assume that adults know best. If this is a carer's experience, it is so easy to slip into the 'Does he take sugar?' situation. This is when a carer assumes that anyone who gets care needs to be treated like a small child. The carer takes the power and the client leaves all decisions to them. So, highly able people with perhaps a visual or mobility problem, have their right to choice removed because disempowerment is what some carers have been used to doing.

On an even more worrying note, there is the danger that some carers might feel they need to have power over others. Having control – not having to ask clients for their views – can make the job seem simpler, quicker and easier.

When asked about the quality of care, most carers raise the problem of resources. Providing quality care will require appropriate levels of staff and facilities, and economic constraints can limit the degree to which clients can be empowered. The goal of empowerment should not be dependent on first getting ideal resources though. A lot is possible even with limited resources, provided that staff teams and centres do have a commitment to an empowering philosophy. Besides a commitment to this philosophy, centres will also require appropriate management and staff development systems.

The biggest problem with empowerment may relate to the kind of past learning that people have had. The idea of enabling other people to make their own decisions and choices, the idea of providing respect to and valuing many different groups of people, is not yet widely adopted in all social settings. Some people still see management as about controlling others. Many people feel that they are being controlled and manipulated whilst at work. The skill of empowering will involve a new and sometimes unfamiliar approach to work.

What disempowerment does to people

When people believe they are being treated unfairly they become angry. Equally, if people feel threatened or that their lives are out of control, they usually feel frustrated and angry. If this anger is recognised and the situation is improved, the person may feel that they have been respected and that they can influence their situation. Very often this does not happen. Instead of recognising the client's rights and needs, the client's anger is seen as unreasonable or as a symptom of their illness. When this happens, the client will experience being disempowered. What happens next depends on the situation, but many disempowered people fail to maintain their anger and instead they withdraw emotionally from the issues that oppress them. For instance:

Case study

Mrs A
Mrs A is 88 years old, white, and lived in a small block of flats. She was married but her husband died ten years ago. There is one surviving close relative, her daughter, now aged 62.

Mrs A first came to the attention of social services two years ago following a stroke.

Her daughter arranged for home care services to assist with household work and for meals on wheels to deliver dinners five days a week. This seemed to meet Mrs A's needs at first, but Mrs A became more and more fussy about the food she was sent. At the same time, the relationship between Mrs A and her daughter became more and more tense. The daughter reported that her mother was becoming more and more demanding of time and attention and more difficult to please. As time went by, meals on wheels were withdrawn; Mrs A's daughter complained that she couldn't cope with the ever increasing demands on her time and suggested that her mother should look for a place in a rest home. Mrs A agreed that she could no longer do anything for herself and could not cope at home.

Mrs A went into a home some three months ago, where she is washed, dressed and fed by staff. Mrs A is sometimes incontinent of urine when she cannot find the toilet. Mrs A has requested the use of a wheelchair so that staff can convey her around the home when necessary. She also appears withdrawn and offers very little conversation. Staff think she may be suffering from senile dementia.

The danger of disempowerment is that it not only reduces the quality of an individual's life, but it might also result in helplessness and withdrawal.

Learned helplessness

As long ago as 1975, Martin Seligman proposed that a lot of depression in adults and elders was due to learning to give up. Clients learn that no matter what they do, or what strategies they try, they can't influence what is going to happen to them. If this learning spreads to coping with life in general, then the client might develop a general helpless attitude to themselves and to the tasks of daily living. So people who are disempowered might start by becoming frustrated and angry. If this action fails to lead to an improvement in life then a process of withdrawal sets in. The person learns that their situation is beyond their control and that efforts to improve it won't work.

The obvious next step is to give up. Giving up saves energy. Withdrawal from events that are out of control may protect the individual's identity. Giving up on life might be a good strategy for coping, when personal rights, choice and control are denied.

If disempowerment leads to helplessness then according to Seligman, learned helplessness can lead to depression and death. The issue here is whether the individual can withdraw safely or whether their ability to make sense of their situation is still open to abuse. If a person cannot predict what is going to happen to them, they are likely to become anxious. Helplessness and anxiety together may lead to clinical depression. Seligman suggests that the stress of helplessness coupled with anxiety results in physiological changes in brain chemistry. The individual is now in a very vulnerable situation. Depression has developed from a long string of events which started from disempowerment. This depression may not be something that the individual could simply free themselves of. Something more than just choosing to feel different would be needed. Seligman believes that severe depression resulting from helplessness and an unpredictable environment can be fatal, especially when an individual is frail.

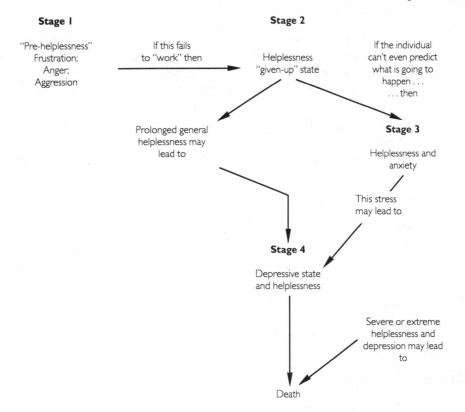

Stage I

"Pre-helplessness"
Frustration;
Anger;
Aggression

If this fails
to "work" then

Stage 2

Helplessness
"given-up" state

If the individual
can't even predict
what is going to
happen . . .
. . . then

Prolonged general
helplessness may
lead to

Stage 3

Helplessness and
anxiety

This stress
may lead to

Stage 4

Depressive state
and helplessness

Severe or extreme
helplessness and
depression may lead
to

Death

The stages of learned helplessness

Case study

Helplessness and what really happened to Mrs A

Mrs A had lived a long independent life. She had worked as a professional dressmaker and had managed her own financial and daily living arrangements. Following her stroke, Mrs A had found daily living activities a struggle. Cooking, cleaning, organising financial affairs all became more difficult. Mrs A had trouble with her speech and at first refused to use the telephone. Her daughter was very sympathetic at first, rallying round to do things for her mother.

Mrs A became frustrated with her attempts to cook and clean, and was very grateful for the help she gained from her daughter. Although Mrs A was angry with her difficulties, she grew to rely on her daughter, her home care and meals on wheels as a solution. This, in turn, proved to be a source of frustration, as the meals and services provided were never exactly what she wanted.

Eventually, Mrs A withdrew from attempting to control her own daily living needs – it was easier to rely on others. This increased pressure on the daughter, causing the daughter to feel angry and frustrated. Residential care seemed the obvious solution. Reasons for loss of control and loss of independence were never really thought about.

In care, Mrs A did not receive a personal care plan; she did not receive empowering care. Rather, her helplessness was understood as 'due to her age'. Staff found it easier and simpler to do everything for her.

Mrs A has little conversation within the home and her daughter found it hard to visit at first. Mrs A has little to do and little that she feels like doing; her helplessness has developed into depression. Mrs A can predict the routine of care, but she can't make sense of her own future. Why is she treated like this? Why doesn't her daughter understand? What will happen to her? The staff make the assumption that Mrs A's depression is possible senile dementia.

Empowering care

Empowering care will prevent the type of helplessness described in the case study above. It starts with assessing the individual's situation and needs, and then adapting the delivery of care to meet those needs. A personal care plan provides the possibility of monitoring the effectiveness of service for clients.

All interpersonal care will need to be guided by the value system of empowerment. An overview of the issues might look like this:

The NVQ value base

National Vocational Qualifications in Care define a value base that all Health and Social Care workers have to demonstrate in the course of their work with clients. The value base is also called the 'O' Unit. According to the value base, quality care always requires care staff to:

- Promote anti-discriminatory practice (Element A).
- Maintain confidentiality (Element B).
- Promote individual rights and choice (Element C).
- Acknowledge individuals' personal beliefs and identity (Element D).
- Support clients through effective communication (Element E).

Together these values and skills can enable clients to feel safe and to have more control over their own future. The value base identifies caring skills which can empower clients who need health services or care services.

In brief, the elements of the value base might work in the following ways:

Anti-discriminatory practice

'Discriminate' is an everyday word which means to distinguish between things or tell things apart. To be able to discriminate means that you can put things into different categories. We have to put things into categories in order to make sense of the world.

The word 'discriminate' is used in a more specialised sense when we use it in the phrase anti-discriminatory practice. Here, discriminate means to make assumptions about people, perceive people as belonging to categories, so that some categories of people get treated better than others. Discrimination results in not meeting the needs of some people, whilst trying to provide for others, because some 'types' of people are valued more than others.

Hedy Brown (1985) quotes studies by a researcher called Simpson which demonstrate discrimination in the provision of health care. The urgency with which people were treated when they might have had a heart attack was not decided solely on the basis of their physical symptoms and needs.

Apparently during the 1970s in London, people were also judged in terms of their age, their appearance, and their moral character. Elderly people, people who had been drinking or people who might be homeless, appear to have been judged as less worth saving and given less prompt attention because they were discriminated against.

Whilst this represents quite a pointed and specialised example of discrimination, treating and valuing people differently because of their race, their culture, their gender, their age and their sexuality are well documented.

Anti-discriminatory practice aims to identify common prejudices, common assumptions and common stereotypes which are used to devalue people, and deny them an equality of service to meet their needs. Anti-discriminatory practice also aims to identify organisational and social systems which have the effect of treating some groups of people less favourably than others.

Having identified ways in which people can be typecast and discriminated against, anti-discriminatory practice seeks to change the systems and behaviours which discriminate. An understanding of the law on discrimination is vital here. Check your knowledge with a text covering Mandatory Unit 1, Element 3.

Anti-discrimination is not about 'treating everyone the same'! This confusion may be linked with looking at the everyday meaning of 'discriminate'. It is possible to understand the word discrimination as meaning telling things apart. So, not discriminating is understood as not noticing anything, not trying to understand the world – seeing everything as 'the same'.

People can be distinguished into different groups; these different groups do have different needs. Anti-discriminatory practice is about empowering clients by not typecasting them, by not providing a differing quality of service in terms of how we value people. Anti-discrimination should also involve positive action to actually meet the needs of different groups.

Individual rights and choice

If anti-discrimination is to work then rights must be respected and clients must be able to make choices. Imagine a school, a nursery, a 'rest home' where everyone is forced to eat the same food – 'they are all treated the same'. Suppose bacon was served up – you have no choice, you have to have it! This would be fine for a lot of people who like eating meat from pigs, but it would offend vegetarians – it would discriminate against their beliefs and values. It would discriminate against people with Jewish or Islamic beliefs who are forbidden to eat pork. Knowledge of these issues is central to anti-discriminatory work, but so is the provision of choice!

As a client you need to be free from inequality but you also need to express your individuality through choice. Your rights and the ability to choose are central to having the power to control your life.

Supporting clients through effective communication

Having someone to talk to may have been high on your list of priorities if you found yourself stranded in a strange hospital on holiday. Having someone who can value you by using effective verbal and non-verbal communication might be the key to feeling safe and feeling that you could cope. If you spoke a different language to the people whose country you were in or if you had any communication disabilities, imagine the relief of having someone who could support you to discuss your feelings clearly.

Confidentiality

The right to dignity and privacy is widely acknowledged as a necessary support for individual identity in Western society. A person's history, their medical status, their fears, their beliefs can sometimes only be spoken about if the client feels that it is safe to share them with a helper who will keep details confidential. Empowerment – the need to have control over your own life may often depend on having the power to share information with carers. Most people will also wish to control who learns personal information about themselves and how it is used.

Acknowledge individuals' beliefs and identity

This value statement requires that carers learn about the individuals they work with. The statement focuses on the need to understand the client. If a carer doesn't understand the individual – and their sense of who they are – it will be impossible to develop empowering care plans. Quality care/empowering care will, therefore, depend on all five areas of the value base, and the skills and knowledge associated with them. A diagrammatic overview might look like this:

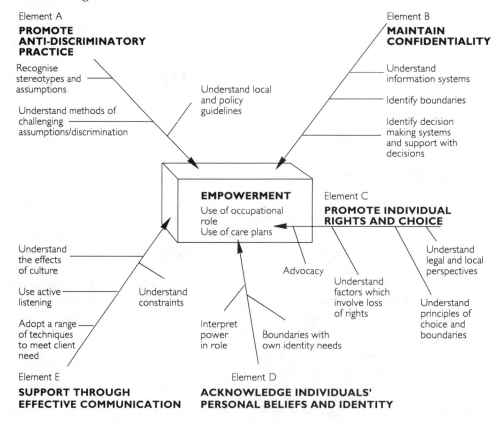

An overview of the concept of empowerment and the NVQ Value Base for Care

Reflective activity

Below are listed a range of statements that may be heard in care settings. Your task is to decide whether the statement empowers or disempowers the client. Mentally place a tick to denote empowerment and a cross to denote disempowerment.

1 'Do not worry your head over such things!'
2 'I am here to do that, that is what I am paid for.'
3 'What would you like to choose?'
4 'I will get a wheelchair, it will be quicker.'
5 'Let me make the drink, you might hurt yourself.'
6 'Let me explain what will happen then you can decide.'
7 'You seem to have difficulty in walking today, would you like some help?'
8 'What would you like me to call you?'
9 'You cannot go on the trip – you are incontinent!'
10 'Here are the new tablets the doctor prescribed, where would you like me to put them for safe keeping?'

Answers are on p. 29.

Providing quality care will depend on the principles outlined in the care sector value base and addressed in Units 1, 2 and 4 of the 1994 Advanced GNVQ Mandatory Units. Quality care will also depend on understanding individuals, organisations and groups.

This book aims to review a range of ideas and theories which may assist with understanding human behaviour in the context of the value base for care.

Understanding self-concept and identity

Reflective activity

The storyline – yourself

How far can you remember back in your own life? Perhaps you have one or two memories of life before the age of six or seven, probably you have quite a few memories of life between the ages of eight and eleven, and perhaps a clear idea of your own history since the age of twelve.

So how good has life been for you? How happy are the memories that you have? Think about your life, what things have given you satisfaction; what things have made you unhappy; how do you feel now? Analyse your feelings using the graph below – put your own line in – at least in imagination.

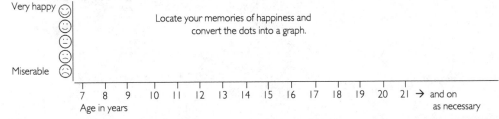

Design your own graph, map your own biography. Where do you think the storyline of yourself will go in the future? What will influence happiness?

Can you imagine something of your past – something of your future? If you can then there is a you, a self who has these experiences, a self that continues forward as time moves on.

Many people don't stop to think about 'self', it's just there. For many people this lack of analysis may hide a simple set of assumptions about self.

The Ghost in the Machine

One very common European belief is that our bodies are like very complicated machines, but the machine is controlled by a 'mind'. Mind and body are separate, the mind being like a person who sits at the control centre of the body. This belief is called a Cartesian view and it is traced back to the philosopher, Descartes (1596–1650), who analysed human beings into three separate parts: the mind, the body and the soul. People in Europe had just discovered that joints and muscles worked rather like levers in machines, that the heart was a pump and so on. This led Descartes to see the body as a machine which needed separate guidance from higher sources – firstly the mind and ultimately the soul.

The importance of this seventeenth-century view is that it has become generally absorbed into European culture and may have created beliefs or assumptions which people don't always realise they have.

This belief – that we have a separate mind that controls our bodies – was called the 'ghost in the machine' by Gilbert Ryle (1973, p. 17). There is a problem with the view. If we are controlled by a little person (or ghost) in our head, who controls the ghost? or who controls that person? If there is another person controlling that ghost, then is there a fourth person inside the head of that person, ghost or whatever?

Looked at in this way the ghost in the machine view of mind doesn't explain anything. As a theory to explain our behaviour it doesn't work. The problem is that it may have become part of European folklore and that people still use the idea to explain the notion of 'self'.

A young child might say, 'It's not my fault' after dropping and breaking a plate that

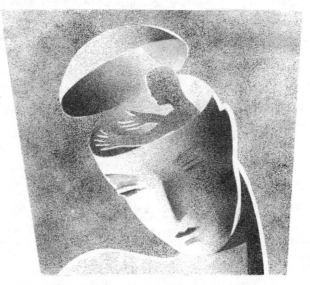

The Ghost in the Machine

they were holding. If pressed further the child might say: 'Well, it's not my fault because I didn't mean to drop the plate – my hands just slipped.' So the hands (part of the machine) are to blame – the mind, and perhaps self are not to blame – it was a mechanical break-down: the mind and self were working normally. The child makes a distinction, based on a separate mind and body which is drawn from their culture.

A depressed person says: 'Now I just hate myself.' Obviously such a statement is very important and meaningful for the individual. Looked at philosophically though, what is the 'self' that the I is hating? Has the controller turned against the machine? Is the controller fed up with a separate 'myself'?

Finally, there are a whole range of deeply meaningful and important things people say: 'I've got to discover who I am'; 'I need to be someone'; 'I have to look after my feelings'; 'I can't control myself – it's just the way I am.' These statements may indicate a separation between 'I' and 'myself' or may suggest that there is some degree of separation between controller and what is controlled.

During placement or work experience have you come across people using 'mind' as a separate idea from body. This is sometimes called mind–body dualism (two parts: (1) mind, (2) body – hence 'dual'). Do you make these assumptions in your own thoughts or care work with others? What are the consequences of thinking of people as being made up of several parts?

The mirror theory of self

'Self, as the controller of a separate person' is a very weak way of trying to explain personal experience, not least because it fails to explain how this 'self' comes into existence. The ghost in the machine view ignores the environment or the social context that people grow up in.

As long ago as 1902, Cooley wrote: 'Self and society are twin born.' In other words 'self' only exists because of the social context that people live in. We understand ourselves in terms of our relationships with others. Cooley believed that people's ideas of themselves were created by seeing themselves reflected in the opinions and reactions of others. Other

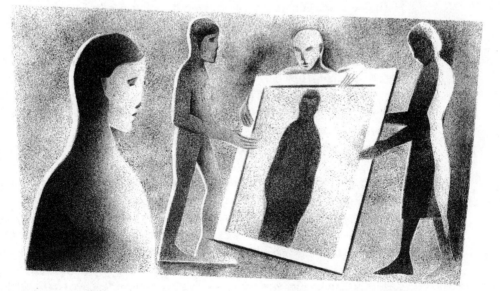

The 'looking glass' or 'mirror' theory of self

people acted like a mirror which gave us ideas as to who we were. This became the 'looking glass' or 'mirror' theory of self.

If other people praise us and say we are attractive, intelligent, sociable, then we might begin to develop a concept of ourselves as a person who is attractive, intelligent and sociable.

If the social groups we mix with value slim body builds, we may begin to wish we were thinner; if the social groups never mention body shape, we may never think about our size and weight. If being healthy – in the eyes of our social group – involves being muscular, we may evaluate ourselves as needing to be heavier and stronger. The way we learn about self depends on the attitudes and values that exist in our cultural context. According to Cooley, what we understand as self is dependent on what is reflected to us from others.

The story of the ugly duckling

Once upon a time, on a pond not far away, lived a society of swans, ducks and other wildfowl. Cygnet, the heroine of this story was an orphan, her parents having been poisoned through eating lead fishing weights. Cygnet was lonely and desperately wanted to be accepted into the fly-catching and dabbling games that all the waterfowl enjoyed. Whenever Cygnet tried to join in with the ducks, they chased her away saying: 'You're too big to be with us, you don't look like us' [at this time there were no NVQs or GNVQs in Caring available on the pond and none of the wildfowl had heard of the 'O' Unit]. When Cygnet tried to join in with the swans, they chased her away saying: 'You're stupid – incompetent, and you don't belong with us, you're an "SEP" [somebody else's problem]'.

Dejected and depressed, Cygnet went to her local pond social services, but all they could offer her was bed and breakfast in a lonely clump of weeds where she had to spend the winter. While there, she reflected on how inadequate she was, and decided that the rest of the pond was right to keep her there out of the way, so that her ugliness didn't cause any offence to others. Eventually, Cygnet came to accept her role on the pond – at least she didn't have to share her worms, water beetles and other insects, and she did have her own clump of weeds.

Then something terrible happened. A whole flock of swans came by and destroyed her self concept. They did it by saying: 'You're a very fine swan indeed, please won't you join us.' At first Cygnet told them 'where to get off', but as they persisted, Cygnet could feel that she was just going to go to pieces inside. These so and so's were telling her that she had totally misunderstood life on the pond, they were telling her that her life had been nonsense so far – they were telling her that she was a swan!

A thought then came to Cygnet, 'Well, this really is rock bottom – from this point on things can't get any worse, why not go along with it?' So Cygnet decided to join in and followed the swans. They explained: 'Being a swan isn't so difficult, you'll soon get into the philosophy, just stick with us.' Cygnet did, and she changed her name to fit her new identity. She lived happily ever after and was very kind and sensitive to any lost and lonely wildfowl that looked as if they too might grow into swans at some stage. Because Cygnet was now a swan, she was very negative to the ducks who she

thought were inferior, but then there was no 'O' Unit and she had not developed formal operational logic as applied to social reasoning (see p. 74).
Moral: Never rely on a theory of self which says that self is a simple result of social influences.

The idea that people's understanding of self is influenced by social context and doesn't exist in a vacuum is very important, but society as a mirror can't be the whole of the story. The idea seems to work when we imagine ourselves as isolated, with a 'society' on the other side holding up a mirror for ourselves to see ourselves in. But surely this is not how we really live. We are part of society, not separate from it. The 'ugly duckling' in the fantasy story was forced into isolation. Very few people suffer such a fate. If we are members of social groups then our behaviour will influence how other members reflect back to us. We might be mirroring reflections back to others. The real picture might look like this:

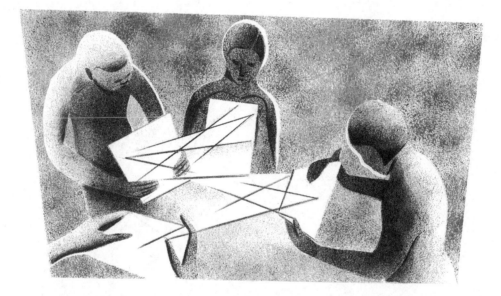

At this point the theory might stop being so useful. The mirror idea can help us understand that our thinking is influenced by social context, but if everyone influences everyone else you get reflections of reflections. We see ourselves in another group's mirror, holding a mirror which reflects that other group – the reflections bounce backwards and forwards. Self becomes influenced by an infinite network of feedback and reflection. Perhaps this is exactly what happens in a sense, but the problem is that the 'mirror' theory doesn't help us to explain much about people's understanding of themselves.

If 'society' or 'social influences' do help to create our sense of who we are, then what are these influences?

Social influences on self

Some of the most important social influences which affect the way we understand ourselves include:

- Our personal interaction with our family or other 'support networks' of people that we grow up with.
- Our friendship networks – the individuals and groups of people that we choose to mix with.
- Our general social experience – the groups and collections of people that we find ourselves mixing with: at work; when we travel; when we go out for entertainment.
- The broader context of our social groups. The experiences we have are influenced by social factors such as our gender, our ethnic group membership, our social class membership, our age group.
- The economic and political context of society.
- The historical background to all the above influences.

The way that these influences work may look something like this:

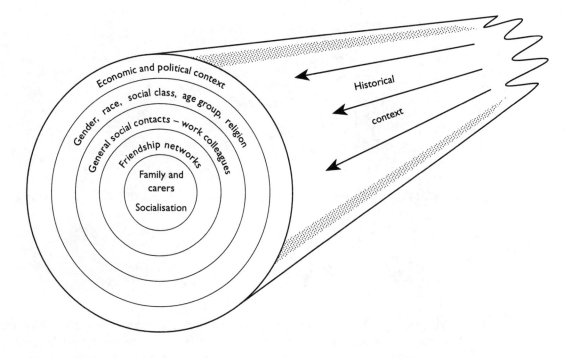

Image of moving in time

Individuals build up a view of themselves and of the world from the conversation, play and general social interaction they have with people in their family or support network. This is referred to as primary socialisation. As we grow older our concepts and beliefs become developed so that we can make sense of a wider social context – our friends and the groups we mix with. The demands of education and work force us to learn about an even wider range of social groups. We may come to see ourselves as being like some people – but not like other people. We build a concept of ourselves based on the groups that we believe we belong to, and we distinguish ourselves from the groups that we come to believe are different.

Tajfel (1971) argues that it is enough to believe that you belong to a group different from other groups for this to affect social identity. Once belonging to a group becomes part of identity, the risk of discriminating against different groups begins. Children from a particular housing estate or particular road may see themselves as an 'in-group' – a social group that belongs together. This group might give themselves a name, may invent rules for membership and so on. The group or gang may then need to define outsiders as the 'out-group': people who are enemies, people to dislike, people who don't fit local expectations, people who are weird. Just believing that you belong to a group may be enough to cause people to categorise themselves and others as 'in-group' and 'out-group', according to Tajfel (1971). This categorisation then leads to persecution and discrimination.

The in-group/out-group theory is often used to explain some of the psychology of racism, sexism, and ageism. People may come to see their own gender, ethnic, or age group as superior to others. The socialised learning about group membership may be at the heart of the self-concept of people who feel that they are superior to others.

Hedy Brown (1985) argues that the situation needs to be understood in terms of levels of explanation. Most people believe that they have their own way of understanding life – their own individually learned and invented way of interpreting the world around them. This is the individual level of explanation. But people are influenced by their socialisation and group membership. We need to understand individuals' experience of groups in order to understand their social behaviour – this is the group level of explanation. But groups don't exist in isolation any more than individuals do! What friends and family tell us is influenced by advertising, stories in the newspapers and TV. These things are influenced by the political and economic systems that operate in society. All of this is the societal level of explanation.

Our understanding of social reality is learned from experience, but it isn't necessarily taught by anyone. Many people try to understand everything in terms of their own personal experience, or their experience in relation to other people that they know personally. The broader societal level of explanation will be needed to place personal explanation in context.

Our understanding of issues like wealth, class, gender, ethnicity, is undoubtedly strongly influenced by broader societal influences such as advertising, economic policy, the law and so on. The question is, do these influences cause our understanding of ourselves – is this the end of the story?

The problem with seeing our self-concept as made by social influences is that it ignores our human abilities to perceive, interpret and understand. Seeing self as an outcome of 'social forces' or social influences seems to reduce people to objects. People interact with the social factors that influence them, they ignore some pressures but quickly respond to others. Sometimes two children will grow up with the same social circumstances – the same environment – yet they will develop quite different views of themselves. So what else is involved?

One view is that 'society makes people into something'. Another view is that people learn to be the way they are because they are influenced by society.

The two views are really very separate: the first view sees people as if they were made of plasticine. Society moulds the person into shape and the person has no say whatsoever.

The problem with this view is that if this were true we would only have to find a way of controlling the family, the economy, relationships, etc., and we could produce people with any views and any behaviour we wanted.

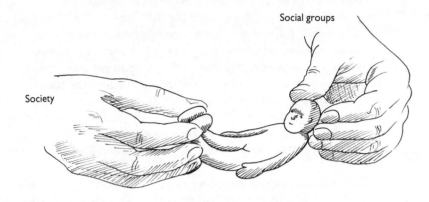

Only plasticine people are moulded by social influences!

Many famous writers have argued that this is possible. Governments such as the Soviet Union, under Stalin, tried to produce people to fit the model they wanted. B.F. Skinner (1902–1990) argued that learning theory could be used to produce socially desirable behaviours – right across the whole of a country or society. While there may still be a few people who believe this, it seems that there is little evidence of any total control system working. People can be manipulated by threats and incentives, but human behaviour seems to be more complicated than just a simple outcome of social pressures. What complicates it? The answer is that people interact with social pressures – they learn.

Imagining a 'me'

'Self' may be strongly influenced by a learning process. What is this learning process? One of the first theories to try and explain this learning of self was G.H. Mead's 1934 theory. People need to be able to predict and make sense of the situations they find themselves in. To begin with, children have to guess how others react and what they will do in situations. According to Mead, the child's experience in trying to understand other people's behaviour leads the child to invent ideas of average people – or generalised characters. Mead called these characters 'generalised others'.

Speculation

Have you noticed how some children (often three to eight years old) have imaginary friends – a pet lion, a person who lives in a crack in the bedroom wall, the 'drawer people' and so on.

These imaginary friends can be told off, can guide the child as to what to do and so on. One idea is that these imaginary people are inventions which help the child to begin to make sense of the way people actually behave. By having an imaginary person, the child can experiment in imagination with social rules and relationships. Imaginary people could be a bit like 'generalised others'.

Because children learn to invent general characters in imagination, it is not long before they can invent an idea of 'self'. Mead used the idea of 'I' and 'me' to explain what happens. The inventor is 'I'; the child who is doing the thinking is 'I'. What they imagine is a separate imaginary person who becomes 'me'. So 'me' is an invention of our minds, based on what we have learned about the way people behave socially. 'I' does the inventing, 'me' is the outcome of the process. We invent a 'me' or a 'self' in order to help us predict how others will react to us.

Play enables children to get to know one another and to begin to behave socially. Play helps children to begin to guess at what people expect from them. By the time children can play games with rules, the child will need to have imagined a 'self' or a 'me' which can fit in with the social rules!

Key consequences of this theory

> The idea of self is an invention, an invention which is based on what we learn to predict from our experience with others.

Mead's theory helps to explain the 'ghost in the machine view of self'. We can imagine a 'self' which helps to explain our social experience. Because we have an imaginary 'me', and we think about this 'me' in order to work out how to behave, it's only one step further to imagining that this 'me' is a separate person living inside us!

Reflective activity

Uses of our imagined 'me' or 'self'

1 Imagine you have an interview for a job – you may feel tense and worried – how can you reduce your worries? Most people try to imagine themselves being interviewed. By imagining a self who knows what to say, we get ourselves into a frame of mind where we can cope and say the right things. We need to picture a 'me' or a 'self' doing the 'right' things.

2 You have to work with a client who is sometimes rude and aggressive! They may make you tense. How can you prepare for this encounter?

Answer: Imagine yourself coping with it. If you can imagine a self saying and doing the right things, then you are more likely to cope than if you can't imagine a 'me' or a 'self' at work.

How do you feel about your imagined 'self', or 'me'? This will depend on social influences according to Mead. As in the mirror theory, you won't be able to imagine yourself doing well at an interview if you've been constantly told you are bad at it. The self that you can imagine has to be supported by evidence from other people. To believe in a self that is good at interviews you would need feedback from others that you are good at interviews. If people give you verbal and non-verbal messages that they think highly of you, if you get congratulated on the way you cope with stress and aggression – then you have evidence that you can use to support your imagination of a successful self. If the reverse happens it's hard to imagine a self who is effective.

So, in Mead's theory, self is invented or imagined but it isn't a fantasy, it has to be based on evidence from other people – it is strongly affected by social influences. We create a self to help us understand and predict our place in the social world that we find ourself in. Our self isn't given to us by society, or given to us by other people. We invent an idea or concept of 'self' but our invention has to fit with our social experience, and is invented from that social experience and learning.

This theory of 'self' may at first look like a final answer but the theory still leaves a lot of real life puzzles unanswered. This 'self' or 'me' which is imagined, sounds as if it is a permanent 'thing'. It sounds as if we all just have one 'self' – one understanding of who we are, how we should act and what we should do.

The only problem is that there is a lot of evidence that this is not how people really behave or act. Some of the earliest research which casts doubt on the idea of a consistent self was conducted by Hartshorne and May in 1930. These researchers asked children questions about what was right and wrong. They also observed what children really did at school, in the playground, after school and so on.

What Hartshorne and May found was that children were not consistent in what they said and what they did. Children also behaved differently in one real situation as compared to another. Hartshorne and May failed to identify any general quality of moral behaviour which governed what happened. The social context of the children seemed more important.

Minard (1952) studied miners in West Virginia, USA. The study explored racist behaviour amongst white miners. Instead of finding that a certain percentage of people held racist views, Minard found that a majority of people changed their behaviour depending on where they were at the time. Roughly 20 per cent of miners held racist views both at work and socially. Twenty per cent of the miners were not racist and 60 per cent of miners held racist views when not at work, but changed their behaviour when they went to work underground!

There is a whole series of research by Sherif and others (1953, 1955 and 1961) which shows how boys constantly altered their views of others depending on what team or group they were in at the time.

It seems that people often fail to be definite and consistent in the way they understand their own social obligations and actions. Perhaps we develop an idea of 'self' – yet this self is not the whole picture when it comes to understanding attitudes and social behaviour. Although we imagine 'selves' to help us predict and cope with other people, it seems that this self does not always result in logically consistent behaviour. Goffman (1971) offers an explanation. Self is not just one permanent invention. Self is constantly adapted and altered depending on the social context and social role that a person finds themselves playing.

The concept of social role

The idea of 'role' comes from play acting. Characters take on identities or roles when they act a character in a play. The role is everything that character is supposed to do and say while they are on display on the stage. As soon as the actor is out of view they can drop the act and behave as their 'normal self'; as long as they are in view they must stick to the part they have been given and do everything as the audience would expect them to do 'in their role'.

Goffman adapted the idea of play acting to make the point that real social life is often like performing in a play. For example, take the job of being a carer at a day nursery. When you go into the building people will have expectations about how you will behave. The staff would expect you to listen to them and discuss issues. The children would expect adult responsibility and behaviour. The parents might expect standards of appearance and friendliness. The exact expectations might vary but each worker has a role set of particular people. These people create a set of expectations for the care worker to perform to. The care worker may feel bored or miserable, but they cannot behave that way when in their role, at work. Client needs come first and the worker must be prepared to change their behaviour to fit the requirements of the role.

Goffman's idea of role suggests that perhaps people's idea of me or self involves different 'me's'. 'Me' as a care worker, 'me' as a friend, 'me' as a member of a social group. Instead of one self, we may turn out to have several selves or several views of self, which allow us to behave according to the needs of a given set of social expectations. People may only be consistent with the demands of a given role – not consistent over the whole of their life.

Reflective activity

Think of two or three distinct roles that you have, student, care worker, member of a family or domestic group. Thinking of yourself in each of these different roles, how do you picture your behaviour in the following general situations?

1 You are asked to help with a straightforward practical task like sorting out a cupboard.
2 Another member of the group is angry with you and accuses you of not listening to them.
3 You were going out or leaving the premises when you are asked to stay for just another half hour to sort out some details.
4 Another person in the group criticises your choice of clothes.

Would you behave consistently across all the roles or do the roles make major differences to what you would do? How does role influence the 'idea' of self you have?

Self-actualisation

If 'self' is variable, if it's just an invention based on our social experience, does this provide a satisfactory explanation? Will this do as a final theory? The problem some people now have is that multiple selves may not feel right. Even if we do change and alter what we do in different situations, we like to think that we are the same person. The idea that we are lots of different people – different 'me's' isn't very satisfactory.

Carl Rogers (1902–1987) provides a view of self that may help with this difficulty. Rogers adopted a belief that was popular in the 1950s and 60s, that living creatures or organisms have an inbuilt tendency to 'self-actualise'. Self-actualise means that animals or humans biologically try to become as healthy and as effective as they can be – they try to fulfil their biological potential. When talking about humans this biological potential includes much more than physical growth and health – it includes mental fulfilment and even what some people might call spiritual fulfilment. Achieving what might be 'in you' to be capable of achieving. Self-actualisation involves a process of developing our idea of 'self' even more closely to our idea of an ideal self – the person we would like to be. Our idea of self is influenced by society – it is influenced and may change because of the roles we find ourselves playing in life. But the point is that self has a purpose. This purpose is more than just learning how to cope socially. The purpose is a constant process of growth or development towards self-actualisation. Self-actualisation is the goal that might unite the separate experiences of 'me', which otherwise might make life seem pointless and empty.

Social influences on self-concept are important in a special way; according to Rogers, all people have a need for 'positive regard'. As a child we need to feel liked, we need respect and sympathy from others – usually from parents. As adults, this need grows into a need for 'positive self regard'. To begin with we need to know that others 'like' us; in time we have to like the self we think we have become. The big problem is that as children, we might learn that being liked depends on doing things to please others.

Being respected, given affection, being loved, might depend on being 'well behaved', on pleasing parents or care givers. Children might learn that being thought well of depends on their achievement. 'If you pass your exams we will buy you a bike/car'; 'You don't want to be like your sister/brother, they're nobody – they didn't achieve anything'; 'You're good – you never make a fuss, you're better than the others because you're quiet.'

Rogers believed that children often learned that getting love, respect, etc., or positive regard, depended on what they did. The regard was 'conditional' on them behaving in the right way. Rogers also believed that conditional positive regard – liking people only if they please our own expectations and wishes – caused a lot of unhappiness, as people struggled to force themselves to conform. Rogers believed that social pressures to conform can prevent people from self-actualising.

Children gradually learn that they will be liked, and likeable: only if they have the right friends; only if they get the right grades; only if they get into the right career; only if they have the right partner; only if they buy the right things; only if they are wealthy, etc. The belief that you are only of value if you perform the right way means that a person can spend their life not really liking their idea of themselves. They always live with the threat of failure; their self-regard might be conditional on constant achievement or the approval of colleagues or partners.

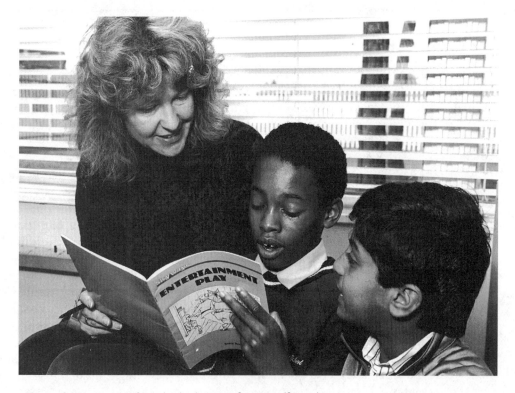

Carers of children need to foster the development of positive self-regard

According to Rogers, the ideal way to socialise children, to educate people and to care for others is to supply unconditional positive regard. This means that a child is accepted, loved, and liked regardless of what they do. Adults receive respect and value regardless of their roles, behaviour, achievement and so on.

The idea of unconditional respect and liking does not mean that 'anything goes'. For example, a child might hit another child in a playgroup. As a carer, you would have to intervene and stop the fight. If you were using conditional positive regard (conditional liking) you might say to the child: 'You are naughty/bad'; 'You mustn't do that'; 'I don't like boys/girls who do things like that.'

All these comments focus on the 'you': 'You are bad'; 'I won't be nice to you.' The adult is manipulating the child's sense of self with threats. Giving unconditional liking means making it clear that you have respect and liking for the child but that you don't like the behaviour. It separates the behaviour from the person. So, in this case it might make sense to separate the children – treat the child with attention, respect and warmth, but emphasise: it's not fair to do that. We can't allow hitting, it's alright to feel angry but when you do you must choose another way of letting your feelings out! This conversation concentrates on the behaviour and not on the 'self'.

Rogers believed that people need to feel 'safe'. That is, they feel that they are valued 'as a person'. If people feel safe then they are free to develop into a contented, fulfilled, self-actualising person. A self-actualising person does not need to pretend to be something they are not – they don't need to confuse self with social roles. A self-actualising person can accept and perhaps understand their own impulses and feelings. A person who feels unsafe might distort or deny their feelings – they may be struggling to achieve goals that other people have set for them.

The self-actualising person is on a permanent journey of discovery, because understanding of self is always open to new experiences.

Coping with life involves developing a self-concept that feels right – a self-concept that fits experience and works. The danger is that we might learn to understand ourselves in terms of other people's needs.

Reflective activity

For example, suppose you attend a job interview. You've written a good application, you have a good CV, you speak well at the interview – but you don't get the job!

How would you feel? You might think to yourself: 'I failed, I'm no good, they wouldn't have me, so perhaps I'll never be able to get into this type of work.'

Perhaps you wouldn't have these thoughts – but can you imagine someone thinking like this? What has the person failed? How have they failed? Perhaps the person has failed the expectations that their friends and relatives had for them! Perhaps the person was trying to live up to beliefs caused by other people's use of conditional regard – 'we will only think well of you if you succeed!' Perhaps the person has failed their own learned social attitudes. They have failed themself, if 'themself' is based on the expectations of other people.

A person who is not being controlled by conditional regard might think differently. Their idea of themselves would not be at risk because they didn't get the job. They might think: 'So I didn't get this job, that's too bad, but sooner or later things will work out – I know I could do the work, I know I'm OK.' If they thought they had been unfairly treated they might think: 'I know I was treated unfairly and I will use my right to complain and get something done about it.' Finally, they might think: 'Well, I didn't get the job – just as well really, I know I wouldn't have been happy at that work. Next time I'll go for something that's more appropriate for me!'

Whatever the reasons for not getting the job, and whatever the emotions, the person's self-concept is safe. Their self-concept is safe because they are not worrying about what other people think. Their idea of themself is based on their own experience – not on the learned wishes of other people.

Developing a safe and effective self-concept is a developmental process that carries on for life.

Reflective activity

Stage One, an exercise in using 'networks'

For this exercise you will need: five squares of nylon or wire netting about 8cm x 8cm square, thirty or so treasury tags, and one large tin of anything – baked beans, fruit, whatever – unopened. Alternatively you will need to be able to imagine these items!

Your task: Construct a bag to hold the can in and carry it about.

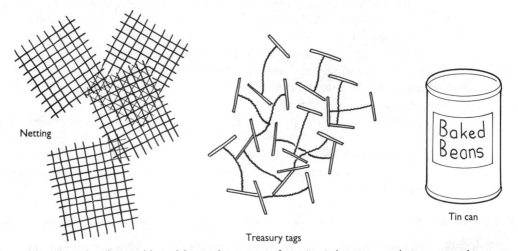

Netting

Treasury tags

Tin can

How to solve the problem: No single square of netting is large enough to act as a bag, although you could be clever and fix up the treasury tags to carry the can as if it was a kind of sling.

A better solution might be to link different sheets of netting together with the tags like this:

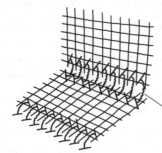

The squares get linked with the treasury tags – the tags hold the netting together

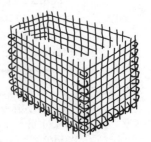

Finally, you can use the treasury tags tied together to form a handle. The finished product looks like this:

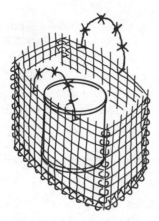

By linking sections of netting together you can create a useful network which works to make a bag.

Making links – a metaphor for thinking

Theories are like the squares of netting in the problem above. Each theory can be used to make sense of some aspect of social reality. Each theory can be useful. The bits of net can be used to carry a can in a kind of sling. A theory of self can explain why people act the way they do. Very often it is better to try and link theories together, rather than just to rely on one idea. Sometimes this is called being 'eclectic'. An eclectic approach means taking the best from each theory. What really matters is being able to make links. You have to be able to see how theories can be linked together to give you a fuller explanation.

Making links might feel like using the treasury tags to interconnect the bits of netting. The more connections you make the more useful the individual theories become to help explain our own and others' behaviour.

Not all ideas can be linked together: some theories are contradictory. Some theories are based on different assumptions. Even so, it is a useful mental exercise to try to make links and to connect ideas up – when you can see a use in doing this. At the end of a GNVQ advanced programme you should be able to make connections between different ideas in different units. Individuals have needs which cut across the theories and areas of study in GNVQ. Working with real people will involve being able to see all the issues together.

Theories of self – an evaluation

The theories of Cooley, Brown, Mead, Goffman and Rogers all supply different ways of understanding the 'self'. People are sometimes inclined to ask: 'If there are so many theories then which one is the correct one, or which one is the best one?'

It is important to explore the notion of truth and ask: 'But we have to ask, best for what?' The theories all say different things, but they are not always concentrating on exactly the same issues – they are not necessarily contradictory. Rogers is really interested in how people understand themselves. Goffman's role theory really highlights issues to do with how social context influences behaviour. Mead's theory highlights the fact that people invent the idea of 'self' or 'me', a view which is not contradictory to Rogers' or Goffman's. Brown's theory introduces the importance of social groups. All theories agree that social influences and the perceptions of others can have a major influence on how we understand ourselves.

What we may have is a pattern of insights, a network of theories which can be seen as linking. Each theory draws our attention to specific issues, or it can be used to draw attention to important ideas about understanding self. Each theory can be used to answer different questions.

> **What is self?** A concept we use to distinguish ourselves from others, a concept which is social and which is founded on social influences (Cooley).
>
> **Why do we develop a concept of self?** Because we learn to create ideas of characters in imagination. We need to invent a character of 'me' in order to understand social situations (Mead).

Is there only one self per person? Not if we focus on the way people behave. Roles mean that the same person will behave quite differently in the social judgements they make when they are in different settings (links with Brown and Goffman). But if we focus on the way people understand themselves, then according to Rogers, a self-actualising person will have a concept of themselves where they can accept the impact of roles without believing that their core self or 'real self' is challenged. They can be open to their different feelings and behaviour in different situations, but still feel they are being true to a 'real self'. So there may not be one 'self' which dictates our actions – but we may have a sense of a single real self.

Perhaps the theories form a network of explanation – each theory might add to our insight and understanding. We don't have to ask which is true or which is best – they may all have their value.

It can be very useful to link theories to create a broader network or framework of explanation. The mental work involved in doing this can lead to useful insights and learning. Experimenting with using concepts such as 'social influences', 'self-actualisation', 'self as reflected by others', 'imagined me' and so on, can lead to deep learning about ourselves. These concepts give us new tools with which to analyse our history. If we can analyse our history, we may be better prepared to analyse and evaluate our present situation.

Evidence opportunity

Analysing self

One of the simplest ideas to encourage understanding of ourselves is the 'Johari Window'. The Johari Window was invented by Joseph Luft and Harry Ingham (1970): 'Jo' comes from Joseph and 'Hari' from Harry! They used their names to label the idea.

There are four areas in Johari Windows. Your task is to think of things about your life and about yourself that fit into the first column: 'Things I know about myself'. How much of this is known by other people? Divide up the details to fit the two cells: 'Things other people know about me' and 'Things other people don't know about me'.

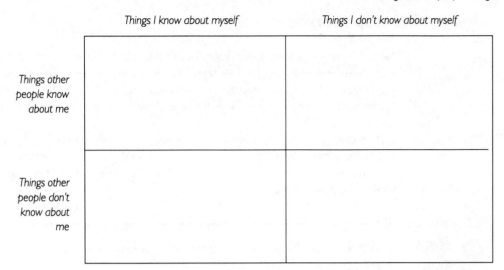

	Things I know about myself	Things I don't know about myself
Things other people know about me		
Things other people don't know about me		

Johari windows

The detail that people can analyse might fit a pattern something like this:

	Things other people know about me	
Things other people know about me	Get on well with my friends. Live with a family. Like pet animals. Learning to drive. Enjoy parties. My gender and race. Political beliefs.	Seen as very able and skilled at work/study. Seen as a happy person, a person that can. cope with anything.
Things other people don't know about me	Feel anxious about my work. Not really happy with my life. Don't always enjoy parties. Have strong feelings about what's wrong with society.	Hidden–unconscious?

Things I know about myself   *Things I don't know about myself*

Lastly, what kinds of impressions do other people have of you? If you are working with a social group, you could ask them for feedback on how they see you. This information goes in the 'Things I don't know about myself' cell. There may be some things that we don't know and neither do others – things about our biology, the way our emotions work, whether we are slow to get angry or more likely to flare up than other people.

Things which are unknown and may be unconscious aren't recordable, but the fourth cell exists to cover this area.

You could work with a close friend in filling in these 'windows'.

Using the Johari Window to explore 'self', we can begin to see self-concept as a large area, some of it hidden from others. The evidence or feedback that we need from others may sometimes be hidden from us. Some of our ideas are open to us and understood by others. This area could be called 'social identity'. Our 'personal identity' might include the cell which is known to self but sometimes hidden from others.

Identity and empowerment

Not all writers would agree that identity is made up of social and personal sections. Some theorists have used the term 'self-concept' as meaning the same as 'identity'. Kay Deaux (1992) used the terms personal and social identity in order to distinguish between the more obvious aspects of self and the more hidden or personal levels of self-awareness.

It makes sense to use identity as a concept to focus on what a person identifies with. This new concept 'identity' can be useful in social care work because it narrows the focus of study. Self-concept might cover everything that might influence a person, the hidden as well as the open areas.

Reflective activity

Why explore our own concept of self? Why explore others' identity and theories of self-concept?

The issue comes back to the core caring concept of empowerment. Attitudes to care may depend on attitudes towards people. If we believe that human behaviour is simply a product of some fixed biological or social system, then it may not seem worthwhile to try to assist people to take control of their own lives. If we are interested in the influences which encourage individual identity then we may be equally interested in seeking to value and support others' individuality. Non-judgemental attitudes toward another's personality may depend on our own sense of self-awareness.

Listening to other people is not always easy. Learning that others have had very different life experiences, that they see the world differently, can be a source of stress and threat to our own identity. The exploration of self-concept may be a starting point for identifying and questioning assumptions about people, as well as assumptions about ourselves.

The analysis and exploration of assumptions is perhaps a key goal of Health and Social Care theory.

Answers to questions on p. 11

1 'Do not worry your head over such things!'
   This phrase is probably disempowering – maybe the client wishes to worry. This phrase does not take the client seriously – it dismisses their worries as irrelevant.

2 'I am here to do that.'
   This phrase is disempowering although it could still be supportive. The phrase suggests that the care worker wishes to take over and do everything for the client.

3 'What would you like to choose?'
   This suggests empowerment through choice.

4 'I will get a wheelchair, it will be quicker.'
   This sounds disempowering – it looks as if the carer makes all the decisions.

5 'Let me make the drink.'
   Disempowerment – the client isn't allowed to do things for themself.

6 'Let me explain what will happen then you can decide.'
   Empowerment – the client has the opportunity to choose.

7 'You seem to have difficulty in walking today, would you like some help?'
   Empowerment – the client is asked if they want help.

8 'What would you like me to call you?'
   Empowerment – the client is in control.

9 'You can't go on the trip.'
   Disempowering – the client is dictated to.

10 'Where should the tablets be put?'
   Probably empowering, the client is in control.

2 Perspectives on people

What is covered in this chapter

- Perspectives and the torch metaphor
- Levels of explanation
- How does a carer find out the causes of a person's behaviour?
- Perspectives
- Behaviourism
- Social learning theory
- The neurobiological perspective
- The humanistic perspective
- The cognitive perspective
- Concepts
- The psychodynamic perspective

Part of the joy of being human might be that we can never fully understand and explain just how individuals work. If our behaviour was controlled by some simple mechanism of mind then it might be possible for someone to discover this mechanism. Once someone had discovered it they could control both individuals and society; perhaps our thoughts would become 'programmed'! Perhaps the reason that no one has ever discovered a simple effective way of permanently controlling everyone is because such a simple answer doesn't exist.

Human motivation, the causes of our behaviour, may be not only complex. In the end it may turn out that a lot of human behaviour can be explained, but not predicted. Behaviour may not be predictable because it is the result of a chaotic system. The modern scientific principles of chaos theory (James Gleick, 1987) may provide a better basis for understanding behaviour than the traditional notion of finding causes.

It may be that there are patterns of behaviour which we can understand, in ourselves, in our clients, and in society. Because we can find patterns we come to invent explanations for them. Sometimes our explanations involve the idea of causes. The real answer might turn out to be that there is no easy or causal way to make sense of human beings.

If there is no simple theory of how people work, there are at least many ways of trying to identify and explore patterns of behaviour. It may be worth asking questions and trying to explain our experience, not because we will arrive at certainties, but because we may at least develop a 'working' set of ideas which can guide practice.

In order to explore our own and others' behaviour it is useful to look at the idea of perspectives.

Perspectives and the torch metaphor

A metaphor is an image or description which can be used to try to explain something. Metaphors are not literal; they are imaginative ways of describing something.

Imagine you are in the countryside. It is night time and it is totally dark. There are no street lights, no moon, no glow of city lights on the horizon. You can't see anything. You have a tiny pencil beam torch. When you shine the torch it picks out one small piece of detail at a time – but you can't see the whole picture as you could in daytime.

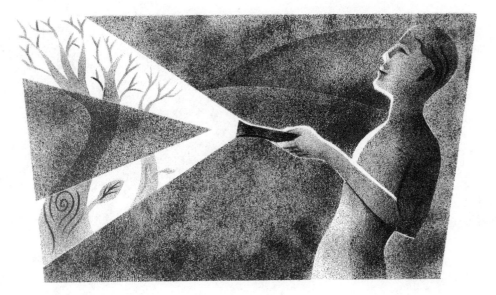

By moving the torch beam about you can work out what is in front of you

As you begin to shine the torch about, so you can begin to work out some patterns. You might point the torch in one direction and come to realise that the things you can now see make up a tree in front of you.

Metaphorically, perspectives are like pointing the torch in one direction and realising what you can see there. Point the torch in different directions and you discover different things. Everything you discover is real, but the things you see aren't all in the same place. If you want to know what's on one side, point the torch to that side and work it out. If you want to work out where to walk, point the torch about and work out which is the best direction to go.

Behaviourism, social learning theory, cognitive, humanistic, neurobiological and psychoanalytic perspectives will reveal different understandings of people and their behaviour. You may be content just to know what's in one direction – this saves time. There are risks involved in not exploring the bigger picture though. What seems obvious at first can prove to be wrong later. Providing professional Health and Social Care may rely on carers being able to question assumptions and recheck what they think they are looking at. Carers may often need to employ different perspectives in order to develop a better understanding of any situation.

Levels of explanation

You are working with an 'older man' or elder who likes to drink tea. You go to take him a cup of tea. Before you can get talking and give the tea to him he explodes with aggression.

31

He swears at you and waves a stick. As far as you can see there is nothing in your behaviour which might have triggered this response – everything you did, verbal and non-verbal behaviour, was caring and supportive. How can you begin to explain what happened?

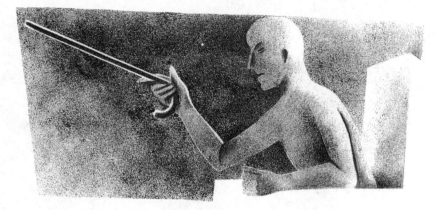

The neurobiological level

When someone is aggressive their brain chemistry and body chemistry are slightly different than when they are at rest. Perhaps changes in brain chemistry might trigger aggression.

For instance, many people become 'touchy' or irritable, or even aggressive, when their blood sugar levels are low (often they may feel hungry). Perhaps the man had low blood sugar and just got irritable over waiting for the tea. Other types of physiological explanations include illness. Perhaps he had a temperature, perhaps he could not understand what was happening due to illness. Perhaps there was a toxic condition in his nervous system. Perhaps thought was impaired by a dementing illness and so on.

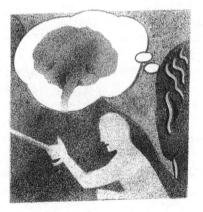

The personal perception level

From your point of view you behaved perfectly, but how did you appear to the older man? This person may have not made sense of your behaviour as you would have expected. Perhaps the older man saw your role as coming to check up on him. Perhaps he felt threatened by you. Possibly the older person's self-esteem was low, perhaps he feared you would criticise him. He may have thought: 'Attack is the best method of defence, I'll keep this person from hurting me by getting at them first!' The explanation for the behaviour might lie in the cognitive processes or in the construction of self-concept of the older person.

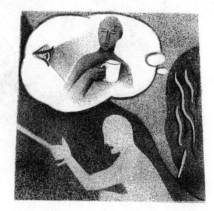

The past learning level

Seeing the aggressive behaviour as due to biology or due to perception may ignore what has happened to the individual in the past. Perhaps this person has come to learn that being aggressive pays off. Perhaps they have used aggression to control other people throughout their life. Perhaps they only get attention and respect when they behave in a threatening way in this home. The person may have learned that this is the best way to survive in care. Aggression may have been learned through a process of reinforcement.

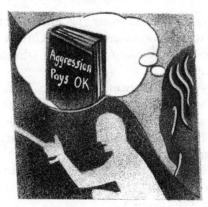

The social context level

So far, all the explanations focus on the individual. But very few humans are socially isolated. A person's perception and learning take place in a social framework of values and meaning. Aggression may have been prompted because the older person held sexist or racist views. The aggression may have been prompted because they thought that you held these views! Sexist or racist discrimination can only be understood in terms of the way social groups behave, and the way individuals learn ideas within different social contexts. Understanding aggression may involve exploring social beliefs. The values that this person may have socialised into might be important to explore. The history of social beliefs also deserves to be studied.

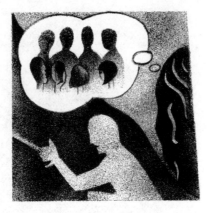

Which perspective is the best one? Many people in care would say that this is a silly question. Each of the ways of explaining the aggression explain something of what might have happened – but all of the perspectives could be right. All of the interpretations could be happening. The person may have been brought up to discriminate against people like you; they may have learned that aggression is the only way to get respect; they may feel threatened by you because you belong to a group that they don't understand. They may be ill and unable to stop themselves from expressing thoughts that they could have normally controlled. All the perspectives work if you want to explore them.

How does a carer find out the cause of a person's behaviour?

There are many different ideas on this question but many people would answer: 'You don't.' 'Cause' is not always a useful concept in care.

The first problem with 'cause' is deciding what level of 'cause' you would like to talk about, for example:

- An eighteen-year-old woman is in hospital with her leg in traction. This situation was caused by a force which resulted in broken bones.
- This force was caused by the woman being hit by a car in a road accident.
- The road traffic accident was caused by the person wandering off the pavement into the road without looking.
- The cause of the person wandering into the road can be explained by the fact that their normal perceptual abilities were suppressed by a neurological condition (in plain English, they were 'drunk').
- The intake of alcohol was caused by the individual's lowered self-esteem which made them want to get drunk (use of alcohol was a culturally acceptable behaviour available to the individual).
- The loss of self-esteem was caused by an argument and dispute with a partner.
- The argument was caused by differing perceptions of social role and gender role behaviour held by the two people.

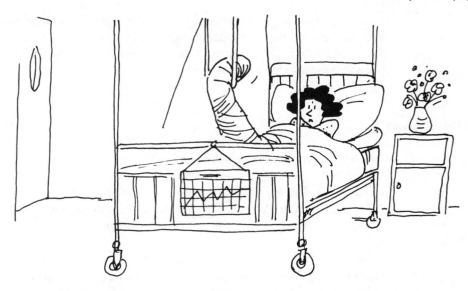

- The different perceptions were caused by slight differences in the cultural values adopted by each person.
- The different cultural values were caused by historical processes operating in society over the last three or four decades.
- The response of getting drunk when self-esteem is low was learned in relation to the person's past social context.
- The availability of alcohol is caused by cultural customs which have their roots in the history of culture.

So what would you like the 'cause' to be? Pick all of these and the explanation gets as big as life itself. Go for just one level and you have missed out on something.

Finding 'the cause' may not be about finding ultimate answers. Most professionals are just interested in the bit that links with their practical work. For instance:

- The surgeon treating the fractured bones need only be interested in the outcomes of the impact.
- The road traffic engineer need only be concerned with how people fall into the road if there are no barriers to stop them.
- Local politicians might be mainly concerned with licensing regulations and traffic regulations.
- Sociologists might concentrate on explaining social role, social contexts and the historical and cultural influences on people.
- Psychologists might concentrate on issues to do with the effects of alcohol, the social perception of alcohol, self-concept and the individual's interpretation of culture, social context and relationships.

> In care work you have to work with the individual – your explanations may need to take in the whole picture. You may not find 'cause' a useful concept – it can go on for ever!

Even if we cannot find a cause for everything it is often useful to be able to produce an explanation for our own and others' behaviour. Explanations are always dependent on the perspective taken.

Some traditional perspectives used to 'frame' explanation of human behaviour are behaviourism; cognitive, humanistic, psychoanalytic and neurobiological perspectives. These perspectives make different types of assumptions about the study of behaviour and they result in different concepts and techniques for working with clients.

Perspectives

Perspectives are more than just theories. Theories offer ways of understanding people; very often it is possible to combine theories to get a better understanding. See, for example, the networks exercise, p. 24. Perspectives cannot always be combined or made to add up in the same way. Perspectives have different rules for what counts as evidence – they are systems of thought rather than simple explanations. There is no way of disproving a perspective.

Theories get abandoned if the evidence goes against them, but perspectives are built on ways of seeing life that are deeply rooted in assumptions. No simple discovery or set of evidence can overturn a perspective.

Perspective means the way things are seen. Perspectives on human behaviour are literally ways of seeing or understanding people. Perspectives are like goggles that we put on to see behaviour in different ways. From the caring viewpoint, we may be able to learn something by using each perspective. Each perspective also has its built-in limitations and assumptions. It may be an important skill to be able to take off one set of goggles and look again through another set.

The most important thing is to recognise that there are different ways of explaining behaviour. There are different assumptions that other people make when they attempt to explain clients' behaviour.

In summary
Perspectives need to be identified when attempting to explain clients' behaviour because:
1 It is important to recognise assumptions that are made when carers try to explain what clients do.
2 It is important to explore our own assumptions about client behaviour.
3 In terms of developing our own mental skills, it is important to distinguish between perspectives which are like systems of thought and theories which are ways of explaining behaviour.

Behaviourism

The term 'behaviourism' implies: 'to study only the behaviour of humans or animals.' Behaviourists believe that the clearest and most scientific answers to understanding human needs can be found by studying behaviour. Studying behaviour means watching, listening and recording what people do or say. Originally, behaviourists did not become involved with notions like identity or self-concept. Behaviourists concentrate on theories of how a person has learned to behave.

Behaviourism fits into the 'past learning' level of explanation. Human action is explained in terms of what a person has learned. Behaviourism is not simply a theory, instead it is a way of thinking. Behaviourism makes assumptions about human experience and understanding.

To understand behaviourism it may be useful to review its history briefly.

The term behaviourism is usually traced back to J.B. Watson (1875–1958), who argued in 1921 that the entire discipline of psychology should be redefined as the study of behaviour. Watson argued that behaviour could be defined and measured. Its study was more scientific than attempting to understand thought processes or internal causes inside people's minds.

Assumptions which underpin behaviourism

Behaviourism tries to cope with the immense complexity of human social experience by simplifying it, or reducing it to straightforward underlying principles. Seeing life through the behaviourist perspective involves trying to see all human interaction, choice and decisions in terms of simple principles of learning. Behaviourism involves reducing complexity to simple foundational principles of 'conditioning'.

Besides trying to explain behaviour by using a relatively simple theory of learning, behaviourism tried to measure and define what was happening. In this way, early behaviourists tried to be scientific. One way in which science had progressed was to find simple principles and then to use measurement to evaluate what was happening. Measurement and evaluation can help to fine-tune a theory – provided it is substantially correct in the first place.

Conditioning – the building block of behaviour

In 1906 Ivan Pavlov, a Russian physiologist, published his work on conditioned learning in dogs. Pavlov was originally trying to study digestion, but his work was constantly upset by the fact that his dogs always anticipated that their dinner was coming. Pavlov decided to study how dogs learned that they were about to be fed. Pavlov was able to measure exactly how dogs learned to associate food with things such as bells which were rung before the food arrived. Pavlov was able to demonstrate that the dogs would dribble (salivate) when they heard the bell because the bell had become associated with the food. This process of 'association' – the bell replacing the food – came to be called conditioning. The bell causes the same behaviour (dribbling) as the food would have originally caused, so the bell becomes a 'conditioned stimulus' conditionally associated with food.

Not all of Pavlov's contempories were impressed with this discovery. Oscar Wilde (a famous author of the time) is reported to have said: 'Doesn't every intelligent dog owner know that!' The fact that both humans and animals learn to associate things together is surely common sense. What made conditioning so revolutionary was the significance placed on this type of learning.

Conditioning came to be regarded as the foundational principle which explained learning. To understand this it is necessary to imagine the science of the 1920s. At this time the atom had been discovered, but it was understood as the basic, smallest particle in nature. Few people believed that it could be split or that there could be anything smaller.

Science taught that the physical world was built up of atoms. Atoms were the building

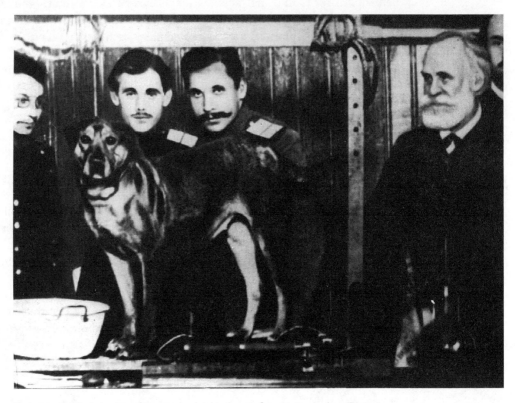

Pavlov studied the behaviour of dogs to develop his theory of association and conditioning

bricks that made everything else. So, if we had the basic building brick of reality, everything else could be learned by understanding how atoms worked. It is likely that psychologists of the time thought the same way about conditioning. Conditioning became like the atom: people supposed it was the simplest principle of learning – perhaps everything could be explained by studying it.

We now know that atomic physics is very much more complicated than people supposed in the 1920s. The story of conditioning may be the same. The picture may turn out to be more complicated than the early behaviourists supposed.

Conditioning in people – some examples

Suppose you eat something that you haven't tried before. You like it, it tastes good at the time; a few hours later and before you have anything else to eat or drink you become feverish, shaky and you feel ill – you can still taste the food. Perhaps later you are sick. Next day you realise that you simply have 24-hour flu. The illness had nothing to do with the food. Mentally you understand it was just a coincidence, but you can't eat that food again – it makes you feel sick to think about it! This is conditioned learning. You know the food has nothing to do with the illness but still you can't eat it again. Your intellectual understanding says it's alright but your physiology tells you differently. You have associated illness with the taste of the food. The food is 'conditioned' with being sick. Just trying to change your thoughts about it won't make you able to eat. Your body has done the learning!

You are out in a car; suddenly you are hit from behind and you are in a frightening accident. Later you understand what happened; it was a one in million chance that went wrong. You know that driving is nearly always safe. Still, next time you get into a car you feel anxious, your heart pounds, you breathe quickly. You have no reason to feel afraid but your body is afraid. You have associated driving with the terror of the accident. Conditioned learning links the accident with driving. You can't alter this just by trying to think it through.

You get a new piece of jewellery – a watch, ring, earrings, whatever. You're going out one evening not expecting anything special. Instead you have a really great time, you impress other people, everyone seems to admire you, you are the centre of attention and you meet a potential partner who is really interested in you. At no time does anyone mention the jewellery – no one notices it – but you think about it while all the excitement is going on. Two days later when you next wear the jewellery, you feel good, you get excitement just from looking at it. You have associated the jewellery with feeling good. Conditioned learning links the pleasant emotions with the jewellery.

Conditioned learning is about physical learning – not intellectual learning; it runs through our lives but may be only part of the story when it comes to understanding people.

Radical behaviourism

Radical means change at the root level – total, complete change. Radical behaviourism was the view that all human behaviour could be explained using two basic learning principles: classical and operant conditioning. The main author associated with radical behaviourism is Burrhus F. Skinner (B.F. Skinner, 1902–1990). Skinner developed the idea that learning is usually caused by the consequences of our behaviours. The idea had previously been developed by Edward Thorndike. Thorndike noted that some actions are inborn or innate; animals and humans are born with a range of ready-made responses to certain situations, for example: a young baby will not crawl over what looks like a visual cliff. However, much of what animals and people eventually do is based on learning. Learning is influenced by the 'law of effect'. Thorndike's law of effect was simply that when we are trying to do something – solve a puzzle perhaps – we learn what works. We learn what produces the desired 'effect'. We unlearn behaviour that seems ineffective.

Skinner developed this idea of behaviour being influenced by its outcomes into another kind of conditioned learning. This conditioning relates to the effect of outcomes on behaviour. Only behaviours which operate effectively will be repeated. Skinner invented the term operant conditioning. His idea was that only 'behaviours' which produce the desired results get repeated. Behaviours which work are called 'operants'. Operants cause people to behave.

If the above paragraph is difficult to follow, part of the reason is that Skinner's way of understanding human action is radically different from most people's usual thinking. To Skinner, people don't choose things, people don't decide to behave in one way or another. People do things because they have been conditioned by the outcomes of their past behaviour! Skinner's idea is radical: it is that people are controlled to a limited degree by associations, but to a very large degree by reinforcers or operants. Reinforcers are desirable outcomes of behaviour. So, people are controlled by the outcomes of their own behaviour. According to Skinner, the idea of free choice, individual responsibility, that people plan their actions in relation to self-concept needs and so on, is all a myth. Reinforcement (or operant conditioning) is the key to understanding all individual and social behaviour.

Reinforcement

Reinforcement means to make something stronger. Reinforced concrete has steel rods in it which make it stronger. If a military garrison gets reinforced, it gets stronger. A reinforcer is anything that makes a behaviour get stronger.

For example, a toddler is sitting in a highchair. Her name is Aysha. Quite by accident Aysha drops her spoon. At first she is puzzled, the spoon has gone. Aysha's mother picks up the spoon and hands it back. Aysha is getting attention and the spoon is back – this feels good to Aysha. So, Aysha drops the spoon again. Once again this behaviour is followed by attention, smiles, and the reappearance of the spoon. The outcome of dropping the spoon is pleasurable, so the behaviour of dropping the spoon becomes reinforced.

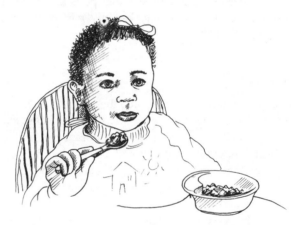

Reinforcement always results in things feeling better; very often reinforcement can be thought of as associated with pleasure. Aysha's spoon-dropping is being reinforced; she likes the attention so she will keep doing it. After she has dropped the spoon quite a few times her mother will come to see that it isn't an accident. So, the mother might decide not to respond this time – just leave the spoon on the floor. Aysha's behaviour of dropping things has been reinforced though. This time there is no good outcome, but that doesn't mean she will not experiment with throwing other things from the highchair. So, next to go on the floor will be her bowl and her food!

In terms of reinforcement theory, Aysha is not being naughty, nor is she playing a premeditated battle of will-power with her mother. All that is happening is that Aysha's behaviour is being operantly conditioned by the outcomes she has received. No one is conditioning Aysha – the last thing her mother wants is all this food on the floor! But Aysha has learned a pattern of behaviour; no one planned for her to learn it but it's happened.

For weeks to come Aysha may keep throwing spoons and food off her table. Why is she so naughty? She isn't, she is just responding to reinforcement. There is no need to bring in theories of Aysha's mental planning, of her chosen decision to throw food on the floor, and so on. Reinforcement explains the whole thing.

What can Aysha's carers do? Perhaps they could try to ignore the behaviour. Interestingly enough, Skinner was able to perform a great deal of experimental research on how reinforcement works in real life. Skinner concluded that partial reinforcement often resulted in more persistent behaviour than getting a pleasurable outcome every time. If Aysha's carers try to ignore some of her behaviour, but have to respond if or when she is very difficult, then operant conditioning theory suggests that Aysha will throw more and more food. Ignoring just some behaviours may be a very bad idea.

Unfortunately, many parents and carers start to think about ways of restraining, stopping, or punishing behaviour. Skinner wrote a good deal about the dangers of punishment. Punishment is very dangerous because while unpleasant experiences can stop a particular behaviour, punishment does not guide future behaviour. So, if Aysha's carers were to get angry and remove her food, after a while the spoon-dropping might stop. But what else would she do and what would she be learning? She might experiment with all sorts of screaming and distressed behaviours, she might learn to constantly act in distressed ways.

So what is the answer? The answer is to understand how reinforcement is at work and then figure out how to take control of the process. Fortunately, most carers can spot this by using their common sense and their past learning; or maybe it's even partly instinctive? A good carer will try to provide a more powerfully reinforcing situation which encourages Aysha to eat with the spoon. That is, they will try to make using the spoon more pleasurable than dropping it. This could be done by providing lots of attention and smiles while Aysha is using the spoon and less when it gets dropped. Using the spoon needs to feel better than throwing it on the floor. Using reinforcement to make Aysha feel good may lead to a way out of the spoon-dropping conditioning. Anything that is learned can be unlearned.

How does a behaviourist approach help to understand other people? Using the torch metaphor, how does it shed light on the complex nature of human behaviour? If you use behaviourism, it can suddenly explain a whole range of issues which are very puzzling otherwise.

Reinforcement – some examples

- You are working with people with learning disabilities. One 24-year-old man called David frequently lies down in the doorway to the centre where you work. David's behaviour causes difficulty for other users of the centre – they can't get in or out easily. Staff spend a lot of time trying to get David to move on each occasion he lies down. It seems that he is getting more and more difficult and takes more persuading on each occasion.
- You have a colleague, Nicholas, who comes to work by car. Each day he parks the car, but then spends several minutes walking round it checking the door locks. It's not a serious problem for anyone – but why does he do it?
- Miss C is an older person or elder who has recently been admitted to a rest home. She often pulls the call system cord to say she has a pain or that something is worrying her. The staff are beginning to dislike her and see her as a nuisance.

Usually, people would try to make sense of these situations by coming up with a mental explanation. Perhaps David used to lie on the floor at home; perhaps he likes it by the door; perhaps he's just deliberately awkward and he's planning all this to make everyone else's life a misery. Why does Nicholas check the car doors? Perhaps he's had something stolen; perhaps he's very worried about crime; perhaps he doesn't trust his door locks.

Why is Mrs C so difficult? Perhaps she doesn't like the staff; perhaps she's trying to get back at people for making her go in a home; perhaps she has dementia.

Behaviourism cuts through all these labels and assumptions. Instead of having to see everything as deliberate, planned and thought through, behaviourism just sees it as reinforcement at work!

David lies down on the floor because this behaviour is being taught and reinforced by the staff at the centre. The staff would be shocked to hear this, they've never wanted him to do that! But reinforcement often happens by accident – it doesn't need any conscious planning or thought. What might be happening is that David doesn't get enough attention during the day. Perhaps quite by chance one day he was looking for some coins in the entrance. Perhaps he was on his knees. The staff may have thought he was in danger of being knocked if the doors opened. They may have spent time persuading him to move. David enjoyed the attention. David went back to look again. The staff moved him on again. David became a centre of attention if he got down on the floor near the door. Now the staff get angry, but David may still be reinforced for being there. The staff may not be able to understand their part in David's behaviour without using the concept of reinforcement. They have reinforced the 'lying in doorway' behaviour by giving lots of attention. It's too late simply not to give attention because David has learnt to lie down. He might stay there all day – he may get aggressive if people just ignore him; ignoring him wouldn't fit the 'O' unit value base. All the staff can do now is to reinforce an alternative behaviour – working on a puzzle perhaps – by giving more attention to David when he works on the puzzle.

Nicholas checks the door locks because he has trained himself to do it. He didn't mean to and he doesn't quite know how he did it, but the concept of reinforcement explains it.

When Nicholas drives to work, he listens to music. He enjoys the drive. When he gets to work there is just a very mild feeling of tension. Work is a bit of a burden – not as good as listening to the music. Nicholas locks the car up, but actually going into work is not so nice as what he was doing. One day there was a doubt as to whether he had locked the car properly – he went back and checked. The feeling of going back to check felt better than going into work; it was a kind of diversion. Because it felt better, reinforcement happened. Checking the locks was reinforced. Now Nicholas has a habit of going around checking the locks. It doesn't make him feel good, but it's a habit and it does sometimes feel a bit better than going straight in.

Mrs C spends much of her day alone; like David she finds other people's attention not so much pleasant in its own right, but a relief from boredom and loneliness. The more she can attract attention the less boredom she feels. Even though the staff are not treating her with respect it is still the case that calling for staff attention is being reinforced. The staff may fail to operate within the 'O' unit value system – they may even criticise and abuse Mrs C. The staff might see this as punishment, but they could be wrong. If Mrs C is very lonely, even criticism could be reinforcing.

The concept of reinforcement is a very powerful tool of analysis. A very useful way of explaining and predicting human behaviour. The key thing about reinforcement is that it can happen without conscious planning and intentions. Reinforcement can occur in any or every conversation. If you regard another person as important, attractive or worth impressing, you will respond to their smiles, head nods and so on. If they smile, that may reinforce you to continue talking. If the smiles and head nods stop you may find that you stop talking or that you change the subject. You are being influenced by the 'operants' or the reinforcers which happen in the conversation.

Observation of behaviour

Behaviourism draws attention to the need to observe what is happening in interactions between people. Reinforcement might be spotted by analysing events which lead to a particular outcome. Sometimes this focus on observation is referred to as behavioural analysis. Martin Herbert (1981) outlines a complete framework for interpreting and working with 'challenging behaviour' in children, using a behaviourist perspective.

When trying to understand behaviour patterns, it is useful to try to identify the role of reinforcement by watching for antecedents (things that happen before) of the behaviour, taking a detailed look at the behaviour and then watching for consequences of the behaviour. This is called the ABC approach.

> A = Antecedents
> B = Behaviour
> C = Consequences

To take a simple example, a five-year-old child throws temper tantrums if she cannot get what she wants or doesn't get full attention from her carers. Rather than label the child 'difficult' or speculate on mental thoughts, the behaviourist would try to watch what was happening. This sometimes requires a lengthy period of just being around to notice what is happening. When the child 'explodes' it would be important to notice what had been happening before: was the child bored, what had they eaten, when had they eaten, what social events were happening and so on. These are the antecedents. The behaviour itself should be carefully analysed and recorded: when do the tantrums tend to happen, who with, where, what is the general context of each tantrum. How intense is the anger, how many outbursts are there, how long do they last, how often do they happen, is there any particular meaning to them that can be interpreted from observation. Finally, what is the outcome?

Carefully watching a particular child's aggression might enable us to identify a pattern or system of behaviour that involves not only the child but the whole social context that surrounds the child. Very often the child may be prompted to become aggressive even though the carers do not realise what they are doing. The carers may lose their own temper, they may lose control. The outcome for the child may be to gain control, or to achieve an outcome which is better than the situation before the tantrum. Detailed observation is used in order to map the pulls and pushes of reinforcement in social systems. Observation is an important alternative to questioning techniques and seeing all behaviour as intentional.

Behaviour modification

If behaviour can be observed and understood in terms of forces in the environment, then some professionals believe that they can devise methods to influence or change behaviour using reinforcement. The essential idea is that alternative behaviours can be taught using reinforcement.

For instance, eating food with a spoon might receive attention, smiles and support, whilst dropping the spoon just results in a spoon being replaced – no special attention. The behaviour of using the spoon is reinforced in order to replace the behaviour of dropping it.

Behaviour modification is about replacing a piece of behaviour with a different behaviour – never about stopping behaviours! If behaviour is motivated just by outcomes – by reinforcers – then it makes sense to try to control the patterns of reinforcement to get positive results. In practice, behaviour modification involves very complex analysis and very serious ethical analysis before it can be used in a care situation. It is likely that much of people's behaviour is not simply due to reinforcement. Other perspectives must be considered before the technique can be applied if carers are to achieve respect for identity, maintenance of personal choice and anti-discriminatory practice.

The limitations of radical behaviourism

There is a strange assumption that people must always have deep personal reasons for anything they do. Behaviourism is really useful in that it challenges this assumption. Radical behaviourism suggests that we do things because we have been conditioned to do them. Conditioning is a basic type of learning that doesn't involve intellectual thought, planning or reasoning. A lot of behaviour is just what seems the best thing to do or say at the time – there may not be deep mental or emotional reasons which explain our behaviour and habits!

The problem for radical behaviourism is that people sometimes do seem to have intellectual and emotional systems of reasoning which guide behaviour. Many people do have concepts of themselves (self-concepts) and their behaviour can be more easily explained in terms of theories of self than in terms of reinforcement or conditioning. Radical behaviourism only seems to be successful in explaining part of the picture when it comes to human behaviour.

From a care viewpoint, the main problem with working purely from a radical behaviourist perspective might be that it ignores the professional value base. The need to understand discrimination and how groups are viewed and valued can't be undertaken within a pure radical behaviourist perspective.

Choice gets reduced to reinforcement within this perspective. Identity is difficult to explain or use as a concept if viewed purely in terms of reinforcing outcomes.

Radical behaviourism may still be a view used by a few psychologists, but in the main, behaviourism has been adapted to incorporate social learning theory. This perspective is sometimes called 'social behaviourism'.

Social learning theory

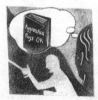

Social learning theory is similar to behaviourism in that it works at the past learning level of explanation. Social behaviourism adds the personal perception level of explanation to the past learning perspective. This creates a more extensive framework of explanation. The term 'social learning theory' is most closely associated with the work of Albert Bandura (born 1925). Bandura accepted the idea that people are strongly influenced by reinforcement and the outcomes of behaviour. He argued though that human thought processes were the key to understanding the process. Bandura (1977) chose to see the idea of habits or responses 'being reinforced' as 'at best a metaphor' (p. 18). The idea of 'strengthening responses' did not adequately explain learning. What really happens is that people interpret outcomes, so reinforcement influences thought processes. Thought processes guide behaviour by predicting future courses of action.

Unlike radical behaviourism, Bandura takes a more commonsense view of human learning. The inner thought processes of a person are affected by outer environmental events. Pleasant and unpleasant outcomes influence thought processes. Bandura introduced the notion of self-concept and self-standards into explanations of behaviour, although he emphasises that self-concept may not be a 'single concept' but rather a series of concepts learned in different social settings. Past learning explains the actions that clients undertake, but clients act on the basis of their thoughts; their thoughts are influenced by reinforcement and other outcomes of behaviour.

Not all 'social behaviourists' would agree that reinforcement works by only influencing thinking (or cognitive) processes. Some theorists like Robert Gagne (1977) separate association learning (conditioning – Pavlovian and Skinnerian and their combinations) from learning processes based on thinking. Conditioned learning can be seen as influencing people on a physical level, while more cognitive (or thinking) learning influences our ability to plan and predict the future. Gagne's ideas are particularly interesting in that he regards basic reinforcement level learning as a starting point which more cognitive learning builds on.

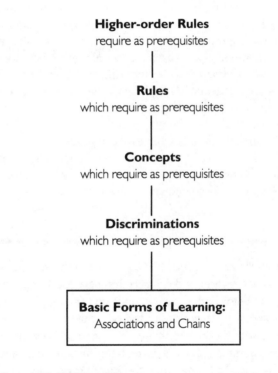

Gagne's model of intellectual skills (1977, p. 34)

Social learning theory acts like a bridge between radical behaviourism and cognitive perspectives. It links concepts and ideas like self-concept with basic learning theories of reinforcement. Bandura's work is particularly useful because it stresses the importance of observational learning or modelling as an explanation of how past learning influences people. Social learning theory stresses that people learn by observing others and copying their behaviour. Most of our social actions will be influenced by what we have seen others do and by what rewards or 'reinforcement' we see them receiving. For example, a young child may dislike having her hair washed. A radical behaviourist approach to the problem might focus on attempting to change the child's behaviour. Usually the child cries, shouts and is generally awkward. The behaviourist approach involves providing attention or anything that the child enjoys (finds reinforcing) when the child stops crying and shouting.

In practice, this behaviour modification approach can prove very difficult. Unless carers have very thorough supervision, behaviour modification can fail to fit the professional value base for caring.

Bandura's social learning theory suggests an alternative way of trying to influence the child to accept having her hair washed. Instead of trying to use reinforcement to directly influence the child, let the child see examples of other children being reinforced for cooperating with having their hair washed. Social learning theory suggests that people learn by observing others – not just in terms of what happens to them. If other children enjoy bathtimes and hair washing, the child who at first resisted may come to copy the others. The child will copy the others because the others seem to get enjoyment (or reinforcement) out of the activity.

Social learning theory makes the same assumption as behaviourism in so far as it sees people's behaviour as being determined by their environment. People act the way they do – hate having their hair washed or whatever – because they have learned to behave that way. 'Operants' which surround people cause them to learn.

Social learning theory is very different from radical behaviourism in that it doesn't see this deterministic or causal pattern as being simple. People live in a social setting, they are members of groups. People learn to perform social roles, they develop a self-concept. Reinforcers influence the way people think, but thinking influences the social processes of reinforcement. Social learning theory argues that the causes of any particular action are usually going to be complex, as it is no good just thinking in terms of reinforcement and learning events. Instead, we have to think in terms of social contexts, individual thought processes, and reinforcement – they all interact!

Reflective activity

The carer is assisting the child to wash and the younger child is learning by observing the process. If the carer and child are having a good time, the younger child may begin to expect to enjoy bath-time too. This isn't the only learning going on. The carer is also being influenced by the reactions of the two children. Their feelings – how much they enjoy working with these children – will depend on how the children behave. We really have a learning system, not just children being influenced by adults! If the carer can get the children to enjoy bath-time, then the carer gets reinforced. Everyone becomes happy: the children like the carer; the carer likes the children – an upward spiral of learning. On the other hand, if the carer can't get the first child to enjoy the experience and the second child observes this, then the whole situation can go down hill, thus everyone loses. Social learning theory can be used as a basis to explore the complex learning systems that may exist in care settings.

Social learning theory and reinforcement theory can be used to explain some events which occur in studies of social care work. If you are developing a case study or an observation study of caring, try to build these ideas in.

Theories such as Martin Seligman's theory of learned helplessness (p. 6) belong within the social learning perspective. Elders may learn to withdraw and become helpless due to 'disempowerment'. But disempowerment may work, not only at the level of lack of reinforcement, but also at the level of self-concept and self-efficacy.

Self-efficacy is a term used by Bandura (1986) to explain how expectations will influence behaviour. People predict how they are likely to succeed at any task and how worthwhile it is to try. If an elder predicts that nothing they do will influence the way they are treated, then they may give up and withdraw. Of course, if they withdraw and give up then they can't influence the way they are treated – it becomes a self-fulfilling prophecy. The way an individual learns to think will greatly affect the way they behave.

Reflective activity

- If you have taken any tests over the last few months or years, how did you predict you would do? Did the outcome of the test fit your expectations?
- If you did less well than you expected, did this cause you to reduce your expectations of self?
- If you did well, did this lead you to increase your belief in your own skills?
- Are you setting up positive or negative expectations for yourself?
- How are these likely to influence your enjoyment and success on GNVQ?
- To what extent do you control the process of expectations and self-efficacy?
- To what extent are you controlled by outcomes in your environment (like failing tests)?

The neurobiological perspective

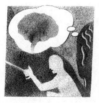

This level of explanation tries to find explanations for behaviour by exploring human physiology. The term 'neuro' means nerves or nervous system. 'Neurobiological' means the human nervous system and physiology in this context. This level of explanation is of major importance in care work. In some care settings it has been fashionable to overlook the influence of physiological states on behaviour. Sometimes, every action is explained away in terms of the client's social perception.

But on a commonsense level, we may be aware of how much our behaviour can be influenced by our physiology. Have you ever gone for a prolonged period without eating? Have you noticed how, besides becoming light-headed, you may have become irritable, snappy or aggressive? Just a lowered blood sugar level can have a major effect on our behaviour.

A raised body temperature can distort judgement and cause a person to experience emotional states which are not related to the environment. No one should drive if they have influenza (flu). Young children often fail to make sense of themselves or their world if they have a temperature. Children will say things like 'the room is full of cabbages' or 'my fingers have gone' if they run a high temperature. The obvious explanation lies in the neurobiology of the child and the impact of the illness.

When care is provided for people with illness or disability, it will be especially important to consider the individual's physical needs when trying to make sense of the things they do. The physiological or neurobiological perspective can be employed with useful effect in work with people who have dementia or Alzheimer's disease, for example.

47

According to Alan Jacques (1988), 'dementia is a syndrome which may be caused by a number of illnesses.' A syndrome is a characteristic pattern of symptoms and signs which enable the condition to be recognised and named. Dementia is not a part of the general ageing process, but a syndrome which may be more common in later life. Some estimates suggest that as many as one in five people over the age of 85 display signs of dementia (see Carole Brayne and David Ames (1988, p. 17)).

- Among the disabilities associated with dementia are things like a loss of the ability to inhibit behaviour (stop oneself from acting on impulse). This problem is associated with damage developing in the frontal lobes of the brain.

- **Aphasia** is an impairment of language which means that a person has trouble finding the right words to express their thoughts or difficulty in understanding the speech of others. Aphasia is partly associated with damage to the temporal lobes at the side of the brain (particularly the left temporal lobe).

- **Apraxia** is a disorder which means that a person has trouble performing body movements, particularly tasks using the hands and arms. Dressing apraxia is a term which means that an individual can no longer perform dressing routines that they have done automatically for many years. Whilst damage anywhere in the brain can cause problems, apraxia may be particularly associated with damage to the parietal lobes.

- **Agnosias** are disorders of recognising people and places. Again, agnosias can occur due to the degenerative processes involved in dementia. Physical brain damage can cause a range of impairments which are not related to the individual's memory, motivation or social perceptions as such.

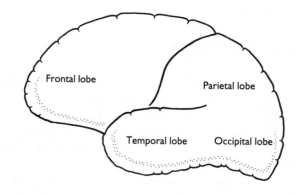

Areas of the human brain

The neurobiological perspective enables carers to recognise the problems of impairment. If a client has dressing apraxia, it may be quite damaging to demand that that person learns to do up their buttons again. During the 1970s and 80s the goal of client independence was often used instead of the goal of empowerment. Usually, independence was meant to mean respect for identity and clients' choice and rights. Occasionally, independence was 'done to' people. That is, clients were instructed to become independent. The neurobiological view would alert carers to the problems of demanding that people dress themselves when they no longer have the ability to perform this skill. Not only might the client fail to achieve the tasks in their care plan, but they might also become distressed when their limitations are exposed. Issues like a loss of ability to inhibit behaviour are highly significant in care.

People with dementia may sometimes respond with rude or aggressive actions. If carers assume that these behaviours are intentional, i.e. planned and deliberate, elder abuse could result. The neurobiological perspective provides the explanation for 'lost ability'. A person with dementia may not be able to stop themselves from swearing on a given occasion, so no amount of criticism or anger could influence them. Confronting the individual in these circumstances might just increase their distress. The client will fail to understand their own and their carer's reaction; they will suffer abuse.

While the neurobiological perspective might illuminate issues which could otherwise be ignored, it is important not to rely on the perspective as a total explanation for human behaviour in general – at least not in a caring context.

Looking at issues like apraxia, we can identify impairment in physical functioning. Impairment is different from disability. An impairment is a loss of physical function while the term disability relates to the loss of a function and its consequences for the individual in a social context. An impairment like apraxia can have different consequences for different people. It depends how people are treated and valued when they can no longer access their skills. If people are respected and valued with appropriate support, then their quality of life may remain intact. If people are not empowered to make choices and control the issues which are important to them, then an impairment becomes overwhelming. The value base for care becomes central to the effective use of a neurobiological perspective.

The humanistic perspective

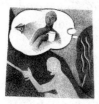

This view operates at the personal perception level. It is called humanistic because of its focus on promoting human potential and achievement. The two theorists most closely associated with this perspective are Carl Rogers and Abraham Maslow. Both Rogers and Maslow believe that self-actualisation is the goal that people try to achieve during their lives. Self-actualisation means achieving a satisfactory understanding of who you are. It means a sense of completeness and a sense of having become everything you needed to become. Self-actualisation involves being fulfilled and content with your understanding of yourself.

The concept of self-actualisation is philosophical and can be difficult to understand at first. Metaphor may help to explain the idea. Imagine a handful of seeds, acorns and plant bulbs. They all have the potential to grow into completely different life forms. Some seeds could grow into sunflowers, other seeds could become shrubs; the bulbs could become tulips; the acorns could become trees. The potential is biologically inside each seed, bulb or acorn. To grow, each seed will need to be planted; it will need sun, rain and soil to fulfil its potential and become what it is capable of becoming. Without adequate soil, light or water, each plant will become stunted or distorted – it will not fulfil its potential, it cannot 'self-actualise'.

The concept of self-actualisation applied to people's understanding of 'self' is like the idea of plants growing. People have the potential for health, fitness, intellectual achievement and for enjoyable relationships with others. Not everyone achieves their inbuilt possibilities. Some people fail to grow and develop a fulfilled sense of self. Instead, such people may become dissatisfied with life. They may view themselves or others as objects for manipulation and exploitation in the struggle to survive.

Like trees that fail to grow, the problem is caused by an environment that distorts the original possibilities. An oppressive society may result in people who cannot self-actualise. An environment without enough light will stop the oak tree from growing.

The difference between people and trees should be obvious though! Trees are fixed, they don't think about their environment as far as we know! A tree can't theorise about the lack of light, pull up its roots and move off to a better spot. People can choose how to spend their lives, or at least people can choose if they can understand what is happening around them, and if they can see through assumptions that may be common in the social environment around them.

Within social learning and social context perspectives, economic and social circumstances are often viewed as strongly influencing, if not controlling, how people behave. The humanistic perspective accepts that the environment does influence people. Rogers' and Maslow's work concentrates on the idea that people can take control of their own lives once they have understood what is happening. A criticism of this perspective is that people have to have some economic and social resources as well as understanding before they can realistically develop their self-actualising potential. Maslow's theory does take account of this criticism, whilst Rogers' optimistic view of people pays less attention to social deprivation.

Carl Rogers proposed the view that people are fundamentally constructive, caring and socially responsible, but that needs for positive regard (see p. 22) can distort this quality. The self-actualising potential is a motivating force which leads individuals towards 'personal growth'.

Self-concept is central to the humanist perspective. Much stress and unhappiness is generated by individuals who cannot live up to the targets they set themselves in their invention or construction of an ideal self. Carl Rogers founded the notion of understanding, warmth and sincerity as the essential basis for supportive, befriending, or counselling relationships.

A friend or carer who can be warm, sincere and understanding can offer a 'safe' conversation. The conversation is 'safe' because the client can review their thoughts without their self-esteem being threatened. If a carer behaves in a non-judgemental way, the client can become free to try and make sense of their own life and environment. The client will not have to worry in case they say the wrong things. The client can learn to analyse their own life. They can work out their own self-actualising pathway without being directed and judged.

People often direct and judge others because they want them to conform to some belief system. The humanistic perspective outlines a way of working aimed at freeing clients from oppressive beliefs. The aim of non-judgemental befriending and counselling is to assist people to become free to develop their potential; or at least to take control of their own lives.

Abraham Maslow's view of self-actualisation is similar to Rogers'. To Maslow, life is a quest to move towards self-actualisation – what a person can be they must be! Maslow's central theory of self-actualisation is based on a theory of motivation. There are two kinds of motivation: deficiency motivation and growth or 'being' motivation. The growth motives cannot be satisfied while there are deficiencies which have to be dealt with. Maslow believed that there was an innate or inbuilt tendency to move up the hierarchy of needs, as individuals quest to lead a fulfilled life. Maslow described his hierarchy in levels as shown:

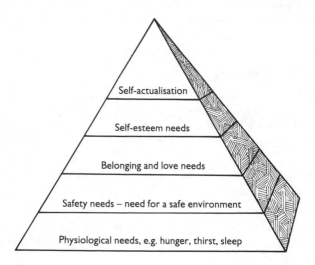

Maslow's hierarchy of needs

Once the deficit needs are dealt with, an individual is free to grow and achieve self-esteem needs. These self-esteem needs are only met by a real belief in one's own personal competence and/or achievement. They cannot be satisfied just by flattery and false praise.

When a person achieves the self-actualisation stage they become interested in philosophical or spiritual issues. These philosophical issues create new needs. Perhaps concern with concepts such as truth or love of beauty or justice. Self-actualising people might become involved with creative and abstract issues. Maslow called these new needs 'meta' needs. Meta means 'beyond', so meta needs are beyond the usual issues that concern and worry many people for most of their lives. Meta needs are not like the deficit needs. There was no order in which people had to deal with them – there was no hierarchy.

Maslow believed that self-actualising people have special qualities: a more accurate perception of reality, greater acceptance of self and others, greater self-knowledge, greater involvement with major projects, greater personal independence, greater social interest, greater creativity and greater spiritual and aesthetic experiences.

The humanistic perspective in caring

The value base requires that carers understand and respect the identity and self-concept of clients. Concern with self-concept and with non-judgemental communication skills is perhaps a vital part of the caring task. Linking the care task to the work of Rogers or Maslow could provide useful 'grounding', a useful foundation for practice. Before adopting a single perspective, it is important to consider its limitations. As with the torch metaphor, it may be unwise to assume you have the full picture just because you have shone the torch in a particular direction.

Humanistic psychology developed in the cultural context of the USA and Europe during the 1950s, 60s and 70s. The 'roots' of the perspective are reflected in the world's major religions and have been around for thousands of years. The concept of self-actualisation and self-fulfilment may be seen as appealing to a particular culture though. The degree to which you find the humanistic perspective useful may depend on your own assumptions about human nature. Thinking about the humanistic perspective will at least provide a starting point for self-analysis.

The cognitive perspective

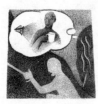

Cognition means knowledge, perception, and thought. The cognitive perspective operates at the individual perception level of explanation. It is different from some of the other perspectives which work at this level because it simply focuses on the processes involved in cognition.

Psychodynamic, social learning and humanistic perspectives tend to present a framework of assumptions which guide us to particular interpretations of human behaviour. The cognitive approach focuses on explaining processes such as memory, problem solving, decision making, perception and language. By explaining the operation of these psychological systems the cognitive perspective might help us to a greater understanding of human behaviour.

The cognitive perspective is not dominated by a few specific theorists. The scope of the cognitive perspective is extremely wide and includes the study of information processing and artificial intelligence. From a care perspective, studies of professional judgement, decision making and the thought processes which support these activities would be of great importance. In order to explore these areas, a brief overview of some work on memory and concept formation might indicate how the cognitive perspective could inform care work.

Reflective activity

Imagine walking towards the door of your current accommodation. You can probably picture it in mind, but have you ever stopped to look at what is really there? How does the light show the colour of the door? Does it change on different occasions? What surrounds the door – are there any cracks, or any bits where the paint is peeling off? What is the view looking back from the door like – what is usually in view – does it change from day to day?

Most people never really stop to look at everyday objects or situations. If we are approaching a door – well it's a door, that's all there is to it, just a door! We are experiencing the world in terms of concepts, not in terms of the unique experiences that occur every day.

Lloyd (1984) estimated that perhaps only one hundredth of what we experience at any given moment actually reaches our consciousness and is actively perceived and stored in short-term memory. Perhaps only one twentieth of this information goes on to be remembered for over an hour, that is, it gets stored in long-term memory. Lloyd's work suggests that perhaps only one two-thousandth of what is really going on around us is remembered several hours later.

It is convenient to imagine that we live in a simple world of people and objects – we see how these things work and we learn about them – and that's it! Just stopping to think about a front door might begin to challenge this naive or simple view of life. Surely, what we do each day is to experience the world in terms of our conceptual categories. We experience 'a door', not the unique awareness of a particular type of light falling on a movable, vertical surface which separates an inside from an outside world.

An artist has to learn to go beyond simple concepts when looking at views, or doors, or anything. An artist will need to see new possibilities, new experiences in their visual field of view. The key issue in Health and Social Care is to be able to go beyond a simple set of concepts for understanding people. The cognitive perspective might warn us not to confuse our experience of our conceptual structure with what is real!

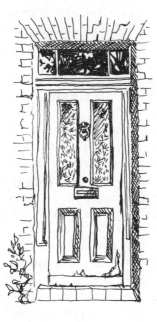

An artist will need to understand visual objects; carers will need to understand people

Concepts

What are concepts? Concepts are mental categories which enable us to categorise and make sense of the world. They are the building bricks of our own personal reality. Edward Smith (1988) suggests that they work in different ways to enable us to cope with life.

Firstly, concepts enable us to group experiences. Grouping experiences means that we can simplify the world and use language to classify it. Without the ability to simplify our world with categories, life would be unmanageable. We couldn't recognise people; we couldn't recognise chairs, tables, books or keyboards. Each new chair would be a unique experience; sitting down to work with a computer would be an act of wonder – we might not link the experience of this keyboard and machine with one we had used the day before. Concepts make life manageable.

Secondly, concepts enable us to make predictions. Once we have classified a movable, vertical surface such as a door, we haven't just labelled it or categorised it. We can go beyond the classification and start to predict how it works. If it's a door then it will push or pull open (sometimes they can slide). A door might have a lock or locks, it might have a handle and so on. The concept 'door' immediately provides a predictive framework which enables us to know what to expect. Because we know what to expect, we can recognise and find memories for things very quickly. We don't have to recall our past lives, 'doors we have known', 'doors we have opened in our time', in order to think of 'locks – I'll need the key!'

Thirdly, concepts can be combined to produce more complicated ideas and thoughts. The concept of door can be linked with ideas like opportunity so that we can think in terms of 'doorways to the future', 'doorways to other worlds' and so on.

Concepts about people or about self will work in exactly the same way. 'Self' enables us to group experiences we have had. The concept of self enables us to identify ourselves as separate from others, it enables us to find memories quickly. 'Self' also enables us to make predictions of what we can do, what we can achieve, what we are good and bad at, how we will react to others. The concept of self can be combined with other concepts like 'image', 'esteem', 'ideal', to give self-image, self-esteem, ideal self. These more complex ideas can give us tools with which to analyse experience, access ideas faster and predict others' behaviour more effectively.

How do we learn concepts? A traditional view in the care sector is that concepts are learned through use of language and are invented within social cultures. This view has been supported in history by authors such as Sapir (1929) and Wharf (1941). Sapir and Wharf theorised that language caused thought patterns. Learn the name of a new concept and soon you will be able to think in terms of it. The Sapir and Wharf hypothesis (or theory) was that all thought was dependent on language – if you have no word for an idea – you won't have the idea!

An alternative view was forwarded by Piaget (1896–1980) who believed that logical development led the development of language, so thoughts and concepts might develop before an individual had the language to label them with. Vygotsky (1896–1934) saw the development of thought and language as separate up to the age of perhaps two years or so. But after this stage the development became interactive, with language and culture influencing, but not necessarily creating thought.

Ilona Roth (1986) argues against the view that concepts are simply created in terms of cultural or group traditions. Roth takes the view that there is a world structure, and that there are logical and efficient ways of making sense of things. World structure has to be 'perceived' or worked out, and this perception is always open to cultural and linguistic influences. So, our personal interpretation of the world is called a 'perceived world structure'. Some ways of classifying the world may work better than others. The way we see the world may be due to 'reality' as well as to our culture and language.

In addition to 'perceived world structure', concept formation is influenced by the principles of 'cognitive economy' and 'shareability'. It is important to be able to recognise, categorise and predict as quickly and simply as possible – this is the principle of cognitive economy. People need concepts to enable them to cope with their environment. A simple set of concepts may often work more efficiently than lots of complicated ideas. Shareability is the idea that concepts have to work in a social context. Concepts which can't be shared with other people are not as useful as ones which have general social meaning. Language and culture may influence perceived world structure because of the need to communicate and share meaning with other people.

Concepts are the building bricks of the world structure that we experience. Different individuals, especially individuals from different cultures, will sometimes use different concepts than we do. This will mean that their perceived world structure is slightly different from ours. Concepts lead to structures. Structures can sometimes turn out to be very variable.

Reflective activity

One way of exploring 'perceived world structures' might be to try this simple experiment with memory, using a story. The story below goes back to the psychologist, Frederick Bartlett, who used it in research into memory in 1932.

- Either explore your 'own' memory by reading 'The Story of the War of the Ghosts' below, close the book, take a break and then come back and try to remember what happened.
- Or, use this story as part of a group work exercise. In this exercise read this story to a member of the group without it being overheard. The person who has just heard the story then has to repeat the story to one other person. This person tells the story to another person.
- Repeat this process until the story has been retold about six or seven times. No notes may be taken, and individuals should not be helped or prompted or allowed to overhear the story before their turn.

Story: The War of the Ghosts

One night two young men from Egulac went down to the river to hunt seals, and while they were there it became foggy and calm. Then they heard war-cries and they thought, 'Maybe this is a war-party.' They escaped to the shore and hid behind a log. Now canoes came up and they heard the noise of paddles and saw one canoe coming up to them. There were five men in the canoe and they said, 'What do you think? We wish to take you along. We are going up the river to make war on the people.'

One of the young men said, 'I have no arrows.' 'Arrows are in the canoe', they said. 'I will not go. I might be killed. My relatives do not know where I have gone. But you', he said, turning to the other, 'may go with them.' So one of the young men went, and the other returned home. And the warriors went on up the river to a town on the other side of Kalama. The people came down to the water and they began to fight and many were killed. But presently the young man heard one of the warriors say 'Quick, let us go home: that Indian has been hit.' Now he thought, 'Oh, they are ghosts.'

He did not feel sick, but they said he had been shot. So the canoes went back to Egulac, and the young man went ashore to his house and made a fire. And he told everybody and said, 'Behold, I accompanied the ghosts, and we went to fight. Many of our fellows were killed. They said I was hit but I did not feel sick.'

He told it all and then became quiet. When the sun rose he fell down. Something black came out his mouth. His face became contorted. The people jumped and cried. He was dead.

Bartlett (1932)

When used in Great Britain this story is rarely remembered very well. Usually about 80 per cent of the story is lost altogether. But besides this the whole storyline becomes muddled and distorted.

Final versions of the story often vary a great deal, but something like this might be left after the story has been told a few times:

'Well five people, five men that is – they go sailing on the sea and they come to an island where they meet some Indians and they haven't got any arrows but a war starts. One of the men get shot but he says he's alright, so they go home and then he is sick but everyone is OK.'

Why isn't the story remembered? It isn't the length of the story, it isn't the two new place names. It isn't even the complicated details with different numbers of people. The story is hard to remember because it is hard to understand.

The story is hard to understand because it doesn't come from European, African or Asian cultures. It comes from an 'Indian' culture from a group living in what is now Canada. The story is also very historical. Unless a person can understand the concepts and the organisation of the story it is very hard to remember. The story is organised around a scheme or pattern of meaning. Our patterns of meaning don't fit with the story. Our perceived world view doesn't fit with the story. The patterns of meaning or schemata, as Bartlett called them, are different.

What is happening in the story could be translated as follows:

One night two men go about their everyday business – hunting seals – but while they are working it becomes foggy and calm. This is very important because ghosts tend to return to haunt the living in the fog. The two men hide when they hear a war-party. We know the war-party are ghosts. This is obvious because: (a) a real war-party wouldn't go out in the fog; and (b) there is no way a real war-party could find these two characters. In European terms – ghosts have X-ray vision! The ghosts want to take the two people with them with the intention of capturing their souls and locking them into the past! One of the warriors tries to find an excuse – he tries 'no arrows' as the first attempt. He then finds an excuse which works based on codes of honour. The ghosts let him go. The other warrior hasn't realised his danger. He refights a war fought many years before – stands in the way of an arrow, and feels nothing. He thinks he is alright, but the ghosts now have a claim on his soul, they take him back to his village. He tells everyone the story. When the sun rises his soul is sucked out of him – it leaves through his mouth. He was dead when he came to tell the others about the war. The ghosts captured his soul!

If you had understood the schemata or pattern for this type of ghost story, it would have been easy to remember. If the concepts of ghost and soul and time had been the same across culture then the story would not have become so distorted.

There are some important points to draw from this study. When people have perceived world structures different to ours – different concepts and different schemata or patterns of conceptual meaning – it is possible to listen to the content of their speech without understanding them.

The 'War of the Ghosts' looks as if it should make sense. When it fails to make sense, people might say it's stupid or it's boring. The truth is that it doesn't fit the patterns of meaning that people are expecting. What then happens is that people try to make their own sense of the story! The story gets reinvented into perhaps a European way of conceptualising ghosts. As this happens the story gets distorted.

So, when people with different cultures and different concepts talk in the same language there is a good chance that the concepts and systems of meaning they use will be misunderstood. Issues like racism are sometimes understood in terms of attitudes or values. Whilst attitudes and values are important, the cognitive perspective would suggest that an individual's whole system of making sense of the world may also be involved. The issue of how people make sense of themselves and others is of great importance for carers. A cognitive perspective may help carers to explore and understand human behaviour.

The psychodynamic perspective

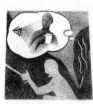

This perspective was originated by Sigmund Freud (1856–1939). It is sometimes referred to as a Freudian perspective, and theorists who have developed the ideas are referred to as post-Freudians. 'Psycho' as a prefix refers to 'mind'. Dynamic refers to energy or 'motive forces'. Psychodynamic – both terms put together – indicates energy and forces of the mind.

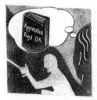

The psychodynamic perspective operates at the past learning and personal perception levels of explanation. It operates at two levels of explanation, because the way a person perceives and reacts to the world is thought to be determined by past learning.

Freud originally trained as a doctor and his early ideas about human behaviour were originally based on the neurobiological theories of his day. Freud went on to originate a view of the mechanism of human personality which created a new perspective. At the heart of the psychodynamic perspective are the assumptions that behaviour is determined or caused by mental systems which are in turn created by early experiences. People are motivated to behave the way they do because of drive energy which is released via the mental structures created during early learning. Within the psychodynamic perspective, every choice, every reaction, every interest and behaviour pattern in people is explainable in terms of forces and systems operating within the mind.

Explanations for aggression or for generosity or caring behaviour are looked for within an individual and within the systems inside the individual. In some ways the psychodynamic perspective is intensely individualistic, always seeking explanations and causes inside the mind of the person and within their past learning.

Freud's ideas and their subsequent development by post-Freudian theorists such as Carl Jung, Alfred Adler and Eric Erikson, are very complex and open to some degree of interpretation. The sections which follow represent only a foundational introduction to the perspective.

Drives

In the psychodynamic perspective, human action is caused by dynamic forces or drives. Freud theorised the existence of a self-preservation drive, a drive towards pleasure and sexual pleasure called libido; and later in his writings, a drive which caused self-destruction called Thanatos. These drives exist within the unconscious part of the human mind. That means that we can't consciously understand or reflect on them. We can only see the results of drive energy and we may believe in the existence of drive because of the outcomes we see. Drive energy could be thought of as like electricity. We can't see electricity but we can interpret its existence when we see the light-bulb light up. Drives were theorised to be innate or inbuilt into human biology.

Id

Drive energy is theorised to exist within the id. The id is again part of our biological make-up. It is the more 'animal' part of human nature concerned with meeting the body's desires without any thought of social issues or future consequences. As a metaphor, the id might be thought of as a dynamo generating drive energy which drives human action and behaviour.

Within Freudian theory, the id is inbuilt but the other two major components of mind or personality come about because of social learning.

Ego

The ego is a mental system which contains personal learning about physical and social reality. The ego has the job of deciding how to respond to the drive energy being generated by human biological needs.

The ego comes into being because the young child (perhaps one and a half to two years old or so) begins to learn that they have to conform to social pressures and expectations. Specifically the child has to learn to control their own bodily functions in toilet training. This is the first experience of not being able to act on impulse, but having to behave in terms of social expectations.

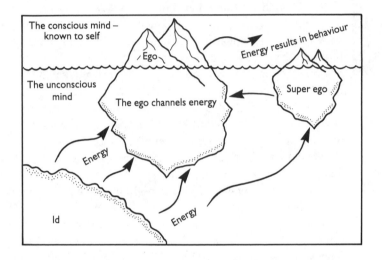

The psychodynamic mechanisms of mind

Super ego

The super ego is a development from the ego, theorised to come into being somewhere around perhaps five to seven years of age. The super ego contains the individual's system of social and moral values. Whilst the ego has to check that drive impulses are expressed in a safe and broadly socially acceptable way, the super ego checks that behaviour conforms to learned social values.

Freudian theory has inspired the comical TV programme interpretations of each individual having three types of people inside their head. We go out to dinner with friends.

Inside our head the id says: 'Go for it, eat it, I'm hungry – it looks good – just do it will you!'

The ego says: 'Fine, but wait, there are social conventions to follow – we all have to sit down first – if you don't do that first, people won't like "me", "I" won't be invited back – the long term risk isn't worth the immediate pleasure – just hang on a bit.'

The super ego says: 'Not only that – but don't forget you're a vegetarian – check everything before tasting; if you fail, I will use drive energy to punish you. The guilt you feel will ruin your pleasure, you won't get away with it!'

This scene is fairly easy to cope with. You're at dinner, you have to wait, you have to check the food, but then you can eat. The drive energy is used successfully – all three little people in your mind agree – no problem.

Next scene: You are working with someone who you find sexually desirable and exciting.

The id responds with: 'Just go for it, get them, take them!'

The ego warns: 'Can't do that, what about the danger, what if it's seen as sexual harassment, what if I look stupid, what about the social consequences – there isn't a social way of going about this.'

Worse still, the super ego comes in: 'This person/situation would not be approved of by your mother/father or past carers. Any approach will be a violation of your internal values – any attempt at sexual gratification [enjoyment] is forbidden.'

The three little people inside the mind don't agree, anything which you do or don't do will be wrong – big problem.

The interpretations of mental systems as people is really only suitable for comedy; but something of the psychodynamic perspective might be explained through these sketches. In Freud's view, the ego runs a daily battle to satisfy the demands of reality, the demands of our biology and the demands of our learned value frameworks. The ego is steering the ship of self through the rocky channels of life!

Frequently, drive energy cannot be conveniently discharged on impulse. The ego has to find a way to cope. This is where ego defence mechanisms come in. Defence mechanisms are tricks the ego can try in order to survive the internal conflicts in an individual's mind.

Firstly, the individual could deny reality – simply refuse to see what is happening.

- An individual could suppress thoughts that they have – that is, they distract themselves so they don't need to think about the issues.
- Repression is where difficult thoughts or images are kept unconscious and not allowed into daily conscious awareness.
- Projection is where the desires, difficulties or needs felt by a person are reinterpreted as coming from others.
- Sublimation is where desires are changed into some form of expression which becomes culturally acceptable.

Ego defences are ways of altering perception of life events in order to maintain inner mental stability.

Besides the dynamics of drive energy, the psychodynamic perspective places great emphasis on the importance of early learning. The exact mental structures represented by the ego and super ego are theorised to depend on the detailed experiences of the first seven years. Personal crises and psychiatric illness in later life are traced back to the detail of early experience in the therapy associated with the psychodynamic approach – psychoanalysis.

Early experience is traditionally described in three stages which establish an individual's personality. The work of Erik Erikson is worth noting in that he broadly adopted the traditional developmental stages proposed by Freud, but added a life-span developmental view. Erikson proposed that there were eight stages of development or developmental crises that individuals faced in life. If crises were resolved successfully then the individual's ego would gain positive qualities which might prove valuable in successfully coping with life. Alternatively, an individual might be left with a mental balance that might prove unfavourable for later coping.

Erikson's life-stages

Table 2.1 – Erikson's Life-stages

Likely age range	Developmental crisis	Personality features of positive outcome	Risks
0–1$\frac{1}{2}$ yrs.	Basic trust v. mistrust	Sense of hope and safety	Insecurity, anxiety
1$\frac{1}{2}$–3 yrs.	Self-control v. shame and doubt	Will-power – control of own body	Inadequacy to control events
3–7 yrs.	Initiative v. guilt	Purpose in life,	Lack of self-worth confidence in self
6–15 yrs.	Competence v. inferiority	Competence, adequacy	Inferiority, feelings of failure
13–21 yrs.	Identity v. role confusion	Ability to be loyal, secure sense of self	Fragmented or unclear sense of self
18–30s	Intimacy v. isolation	Love, sharing commitment	Inability to make close friendships
20s-60s	Generosity v. stagnation	Care, wide concern for others	Inward looking, self-indulgence
Later life	Ego-integrity v. despair	Sense of meaning to life, wisdom	Lack of meaning in life

v. = versus

Age ranges are approximations only. The way an individual learns to resolve their inner psychodynamic processes will influence their expressed personality and their satisfaction with life.

Erikson's life-stage model is not universally accepted by theorists and practices outside the psychodynamic perspective. One criticism, contested by Erikson, is that the general pattern of life crises is true only for European cultures. A more general criticism is that most people experience personal development in terms of a gentler and less dramatic process than eight life-stage crises.

The psychodynamic approach in Health and Social Care

The psychodynamic perspective has greatly influenced European thought. Words like ego, defences, unconscious, are now everyday terms used by people who have never thought about psychology or the caring profession. One reason for knowing about the psychodynamic approach might literally be to check its influence on the thoughts and assumptions which carers make about themselves and others.

One concern with the perspective that some critics have identified is that it does centre very heavily on the internal workings of individual minds. It may be possible to become absorbed in this perspective to the point of ignoring social context, culture, and social systems of meaning which have developed in non-European cultures.

On a practical level, there are major difficulties in using the perspective with only an introductory knowledge of it. Freud cautioned that no one should attempt to analyse other people without first going through a lengthy process of analysis (psychoanalysis) themselves. Personal ego defences are likely to distort our perception of others, and also our perception of ourselves – even if the broad approach is correct.

The main value of the psychodynamic perspective may be to focus thought on the importance of previous life experience and the importance of a client's own internal situation. The main problem with the psychodynamic perspective in a caring context is that it may overemphasise these issues. Practitioners who work exclusively within this perspective will need to take care that they maintain the value base of empowering care.

3 Assumptions about people

What is covered in this chapter

- The psychodynamic perspective and human development
- Attachment and separation
- Piaget's theory of cognitive development
- Understanding our thinking – are formal operations really a stage of development?
- Personality
- Perception of others
- Social influences

The last chapter looked at various psychological perspectives. Perspectives were understood using the 'torch metaphor', in terms of shedding some light on the understanding of an individual.

This chapter is also concerned with the knowledge psychology has to offer which may help us to understand the origins of assumptions that we may make about each other.

The psychodynamic perspective and human development

The last chapter ended with a discussion of the psychodynamic perspective. This perspective started from the ideas of Sigmund Freud (1856–1939). To understand a little about assumptions that could be made about people, from a Freudian perspective, this chapter considers Freud's theories in a bit more detail.

Freud's theory of human development was called 'psycho-sexual development'. He theorised a physiological explanation of human behaviour which was directly related to people's early childhood experience. Freud believed that the human soul could be explained if access to what he termed 'the unconscious' was achieved. Dreams and the interpretation of them was 'the royal road to the unconscious' (*The Interpretation of Dreams*, S. Freud, 1900).

Freud stressed that dreams should not be interpreted literally, but that their content held the key to understanding. The story of 'Little Hans' explains this idea further (see p. 65). There were other ways that access could be gained into the unconscious: the 'Freudian slip' and a technique called 'free association'. The Freudian slip represents those slips of the tongue or pen when we say things that we didn't consciously mean to, which can sometimes be quite embarrassing! However, Freud believed that our conscious mind or perception of reality (ego) acts as a barrier to what is contained in our unconscious. We are never usually aware of these barriers. But a person hearing us might think that we planned to say what came out.

An example of a Freudian slip might go something like this: You are thinking that a serious work task isn't really worth doing but you don't want your supervisor to know what you really think. You intend to say: 'Please could you explain the *aim* of the task to me?' Instead you make a slip and say: 'Please could you explain the *game* of the task.'

You say 'game' instead of 'aim' because that is what you are really thinking. The Freudian slip shows what is going on in your unconscious mind. 'Freudian slips' can be very embarrassing if other people realise what you really think. Perhaps they will think you just made a mistake with words though!

Free association involves suggesting a series of words to a person and recording their immediate responses. If the response has been thought about in any way then it is disregarded. Free association might involve a questioner saying a word like 'tree'. The other person then gives a list of words that come into their head. Words like 'leaves', 'branches', 'sky', 'babies'. 'Leaves', 'branches' and 'sky' are all things which might obviously link with remembering a tree. The idea of babies doesn't obviously link but the individual may have their own unconscious associations or their own story which has caused this word to be remembered.

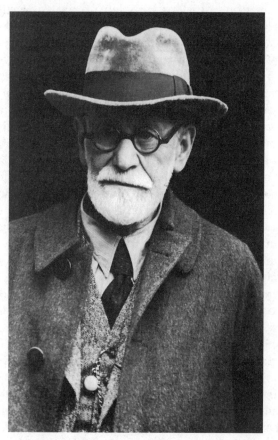

Sigmund Freud (1856–1939)

Psychoanalytic therapy or psychoanalysis involves understanding the unconscious, and was a term that Freud coined in 1896. He believed that everyone should have psychoanalysis to understand the legacy of their early childhood experience – psychoanalysis was seen as 'the key to the soul' (Freud, 1900) and a way of understanding a person's feelings and actions.

According to Freud, a person's psycho-sexual development had five stages:

1 the Oral stage – birth to eighteen months (approx.);
2 the Anal stage – eighteen months to three years (approx.);
3 the Phallic stage – three to six years (approx.);
4 the Latency period – six years to puberty; and
5 the Genital stage, which is the final phase of development.

These ages are all approximate because individuals develop at different rates, some sooner than others, so they are meant to be seen as average ages. Freud called his stages after the erogenous or enjoyable parts of the body which were thought to influence each stage. Certain parts of the body were thought to be a source of pleasure to the child at different ages. The id (understood as the pleasure principle) is selfish, savage and animalistic in that it is linked to an instinctual drive which Freud called libido. Libido is often understood as sexual desire but should be understood as 'life instinct' or 'Eros'. The id can be seen as representing all instinctual energy, which is pleasure seeking and can be found in the human unconscious.

A person's development might be fixated at any stage and this would influence a person's personality. For example, a person fixated at the oral stage might show behaviour associated with sucking – excessive smoking, eating or drinking may be seen! Anal fixation might cause behaviour associated with physiological control, i.e. holding in and letting go. Adults fixated here can be ordered, controlled, excessively neat and clean, and mean and thrifty! Fixation in the phallic stage will affect a person's relationships with others in adult life. The latency period was not really considered a stage of sexual development because at this time the child's energies are directed outward to school, knowledge, sports, etc. The genital stage could not have a fixation because it's the last stage and development would be complete here.

Looking at the phallic stage in more detail it is important to understand the cultural context of Freud's work. Freud's education in Vienna in the late nineteenth century involved heavy emphasis on the classics and science. Greek mythology was always a source of interest to Freud. Consequently in the phallic stage there are two 'complexes' named after a Greek hero and heroine – 'Oedipus' and 'Electra'.

In the phallic stage, Freud believed that children got pleasure from playing with their genitals. Little boys are usually stopped from doing this and Freud believed that feelings of guilt would result from being stopped. This guilt would be compounded by feelings of desire for the opposite sex parent. Freud believed that little boys desire their mother and see their father as a rival for their mother's affections. The little boy also fears punishment by his father should he ever find out. The boy might feel immense guilt, particularly if he wishes harm to come to his father, even unconsciously, because he wants his mother to himself.

In the myth, Oedipus defeated his father in battle and won the right to marry his mother, although he didn't know that they were his parents, having been brought up by others. When the truth came out, he blinded himself and became a beggar and Queen Jocasta (his mother) committed suicide.

The little girl desires her father and sees her mother as a rival. In addition she feels that her mother has already punished her as she doesn't have a penis. In the myth, Electra loved her father and when her mother's lover killed her father, she plotted to murder this lover with the help of her brother and they both were held responsible. A fixation at the phallic stage would show a marked preference in adult life for partners who resembled the desired parent, either physically or in other ways.

Case study

Little Hans

'Little Hans' was the little boy whose dreams Freud interpreted, even though the interpretation was only in letters sent between Freud and little Hans's father. Little Hans developed a phobia (fear) of horses when he was four or five years of age. His parents were at a loss to explain this fear, particularly as he had always loved horses previously. His father wrote to Freud explaining what little Hans had said about his dreams. Hans's father reported that little Hans had been told to stop masturbating by his mother 'or else his widdler [penis] would be cut off', and that the little boy had replied that he didn't care, 'he would widdle with his bottom'. Freud interpreted this as being positive that the little boy would not let anybody rob him of his creativity. Then the father reported that little Hans had dreamt that he saw his father's penis through a keyhole and that he had said to his father that it had seemed 'as big as a horse's!'

Freud interpreted this as rivalry in the Oedipus complex, and that the guilt from the masturbation had caused little Hans to see his father as being a 'mighty horse' and so he had developed a fear of horses consciously. The little boy had also told his father how he wished that this mother would towel him more when bathing him and how he was going to have other children with his mother, following the birth of his little baby sister Hanna. Through constant dialogue with little Hans and the support both the father and Freud gave to the little boy, Hans gradually conquered his fear of horses (based on his fear of his father as a rival). Freud advised Hans's father to tell Hans that his 'widdler would not be cut off, but it will grow as big as daddy's and he could also grow a moustache like daddy's'. In this way Hans was cured of his phobia through a process of identification, which Freud saw as appropriate for moving on from the phallic stage. The little boy saw his father as less of a rival and more of a role model for the kind of 'daddy' that he himself would like to be (from *Three Essays on Sexuality*, S. Freud, 1905).

So what 'assumptions' does Freudian theory lead us to? Psychoanalysis, as a general theory, has had a great deal of influence on Western culture and society as we know it today. Our ideas of gender roles, individual development and human behaviour have all been debated because of, or have been understood through, the theories of Sigmund Freud. Love or loathe it, Freudian theory is seen by some people as one of the most interesting and important psychological perspectives. At a popular level, the 'Freudian slip', 'free association' techniques and development fixation provide a great deal of humour and interest to many people.

Attachment and separation

Another theory which follows on from the psychodynamic perspective is John Bowlby's theory of attachment. This theory is concerned with successful child development. Bowlby was psychoanalytically trained and therefore interested in the importance of early childhood experience. Bowlby also based his theory on instinctual behaviour; in his case, this was primarily concerned with ethology, which is the study of animal behaviour.

Ethologists study animal behaviour from a biological point of view which is based on instinct. They study aggressive, sexual and mating behaviour by observation and they devise experiments to test their theories.

Bowlby was particularly interested in the work of the ethologist, Konrad Lorenz, who had done extensive studies of geese and ducks. Lorenz concluded that there was a critical period of three days in which goslings and ducklings became permanently bonded or imprinted to their mothers, and this period was crucial in terms of their later behaviour. When this attachment did not occur in the normal way the goslings' and ducklings' later mating behaviour was seriously disrupted and irreversible damage was done.

Maternal deprivation

Bowlby (1951) drew on the observations and experiments of Lorenz, Tinbergen and others, and presented a paper to the World Health Organisation. He stated that maternal deprivation could be seen as being the cause of emotionally disturbed behaviour and under-achievement at school, which he had observed in institutionalised or hospitalised children. He believed that children who were prevented, for whatever reason, from forming close bonds of affection with their mothers (or permanent adopted mothers) during the first three years of life, would develop problems of a social, emotional or intellectual nature in later life. He stated that 'a mother's love is as essential for normal growth as are vitamins.'

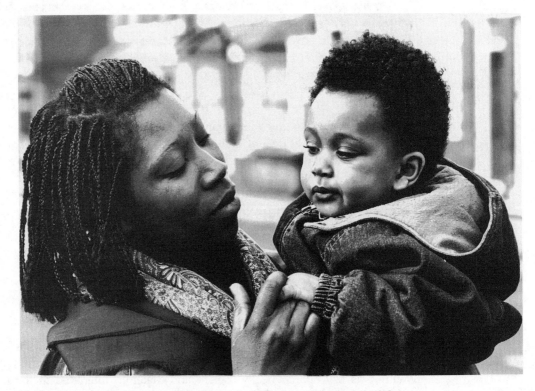

John Bowlby stressed the importance of forming bonds of affection in the early years of life

Bowlby's ideas prompted further investigation of the effects of maternal deprivation by other researchers like Harlow and Harlow (1958), who looked at the behaviour of deprived monkeys. In the first study, infant monkeys were taken away from their mothers shortly after birth and were placed in either of two situations: (1) with a cloth substitute mother, or (2) with a wire substitute mother.

Both 'mothers' were equipped with a feeding bottle, and the monkeys had the opportunity of access to both 'mothers'. The results that Harry Harlow obtained showed a need for 'contact comfort' by all the monkeys – that is, they all showed a preference for the cloth 'mother' over the wire 'mother', regardless of the need to be fed. Furthermore, when the monkeys were introduced to other normally reared monkeys, difficulties in forming normal relationships were seen. Aggressiveness or indifference was shown by the 'experimental' monkeys, males were unable to mate successfully and the females who did successfully mate and produce offspring were careless or cruel as mothers.

Later these results led Harlow to claim in 1971 that mothering is crucial in all primates (including people) to ensure normal development. This claim stood, despite the fact that the original monkeys' abnormal behaviour became reduced after daily exposure to other young monkeys. Contact with others perhaps compensated for the lack of a mother.

Later studies by Novak and Harlow (1975) showed similar results: that interaction with other 'therapist' monkeys greatly reduced any disturbed behaviour in deprived monkeys. We must of course be aware of the problems involved in generalising from animal behaviour to that of human beings.

Even though Bowlby in 1969 and 1980 slightly revised some of his earlier ideas, his basic belief remained that attachment to a mother or permanent mother substitute was crucial to normal development. Not only was the risk of abnormal development said to produce delinquency, emotional disability and under-achievement, but maternal deprivation might also cause what Bowlby termed 'affectionless psychopathy'. This is an inability to care for, or about, other people.

To stay with our 'assumptions' theme, we may observe what appears to be disturbed behaviour in young children, say at school, and we may make assumptions about whether or not deprivation may have occurred during the course of their early development. Bowlby's suggestions extended to things like school phobia, so this is examined in a little more detail.

Bowlby asserts various patterns of family situations which act as causal agents for school phobia in children. All of them show marital problems of varying nature amongst the parents, and in *Attachment and Loss: Volume 2 – Separation* (1973), Bowlby speaks of patterns A, B, C and D.

Pattern A describes incidents where the mother of a child refusing to go to school, allows the child to dominate her in the same way that she allowed her own mother to. The mother also apparently treats the child like a grown-up; this shows a need by the mother to love and depend on her own child, rather than the other way around!

Pattern B describes cases where children refuse to go to school because they feel that in their absence some harm may come to the mother (or father), particularly if the mother has used this threat (of parents becoming ill) if the children are not good!

Pattern C describes cases of children being threatened with harm to themselves, i.e. that they would be abandoned by their parents, and this fear had become internalised, preventing them from going to school.

Lastly, **pattern D** describes situations where the mother or father fears that something will happen to the child at school, i.e. that he/she will become ill at school and so keeps him/her at home. This apparently shows itself in the parents insisting on frequent checks or medication for the child, which are unwarranted in the opinion of the school!

Bowlby's theories owe much to their psychoanalytic base, and indeed, Bowlby's evaluations of cases in his books are done in terms of Freudian theory. His ideas, like Freud's, were largely patriarchal. Patriarchal means that women and women's roles (as mothers perhaps) are rarely given a positive status. Hence Bowlby's ideas of child-rearing rarely feature the father as taking an equal share in the blame or indeed the success of raising children normally; in fact, 'paternal deprivation' was never mentioned! Other theories of attachment, for example, those of Michael Rutter, do show both fathers and mothers more equally as carers in their children's development.

Bowlby however created a lot of hostility in single mothers, because his theories appear to blame them for having to leave their children in order to work. Both Freud and Bowlby, because of their theoretical views, may create guilt in single parents. All the more reason perhaps for them both to recommend psychoanalytic psychotherapy in order to get rid of it. Perhaps it should be available without charge in certain cases!

Bowlby's (1951, 1969) theory suggests that children need attachment or bonding to one person in order to function normally. Bowlby referred to this as 'monotropy' during the 'critical period'. This means that the child needed one care giver during early development. This person needed to be the permanent caretaker (usually the mother).

The view of monotropy has been reassessed by Michael Rutter. In *Maternal Deprivation Reassessed* (2nd edition, 1981), Rutter states:

> There is good evidence that most children develop strong attachments to their parents (Ainsworth, 1963, 1964; Schaffer and Emerson, 1964). In his extensive review of the topic, Bowlby (1969) points to the universal occurrence of attachment behaviour in both man and subhuman primates. It may be accepted that this is a fundamental characteristic of the mother/child relationship. However, it is equally clear that there is great individual variation in the strength and distribution of attachments; the main bond is not always with the mother and bonds are often made with many people.

Thus Schaffer and Emerson (1964) found that the sole principal attachment was to the mother in only half of the eighteen month old children they studied and in nearly a third of cases the main attachment was to the father (p. 19).

Rutter's own theories take into account the diversity of mechanisms involved in attachment and bonding and suggest that multiple attachments can be formed with various people without harm, as long as there is continuity of care as opposed to constant changes of caretakers. Further, that stronger attachments can be formed with a parent, either father or mother, in situations where the parents are not available all the time. There is a need to distinguish between 'quality time' and the quantity of time spent with young children. The quality of child/carer interaction seems to be most important for developing normal social relationships.

Fox (1977) researched Israeli kibbutzim, where children live separately from their parents and are cared for in children's houses by a 'metapalet', or children's nurse. The children concerned were able to form stronger attachments to their mothers than to their principal caretakers with whom they spent the most time.

Case study

Compare the following two stories:

Kam is one year old. She has a five-year-old sister and a three-year-old brother. She only sees her mother briefly in the morning and perhaps for two hours most evenings. Kam spends even less time with her father. Kam's main care giver is her grandmother who stays in most of the day. During the day Kam is given a great deal of attention. There is a wide range of toys to play with and the grandmother is constantly talking to Kam. Kam and her brother and sister are often organised into a group where the older children play with books and music. Kam's mother has to work all day but in the evenings she gives her full attention to Kam, talking to her, feeding her, changing her, watching her play. Kam is used to being a centre of attention and used to people responding to her needs.

Karren is one year old, she lives with her mother and father. She also has two siblings (a brother and sister). Karren's parents are dependent on social security and find it difficult to make ends meet. Although Karren's mother is usually in the house she is often busy with household activities. Karren's mother often becomes tired and depressed and cannot be bothered to play with her. The other two children often fight and Karren's mother becomes angry and abusive. The household feels stressed. Karren's father is often out. Karren's mother is exhausted and she sees the children as a burden. The mother wishes she could be free of the children at least for a while. Karren's mother doesn't spend a lot of time with her. She mainly just feeds and changes Karren. Karren doesn't get a great deal of attention despite being with her mother most of the time.

At first glance the theory of maternal deprivation might seem to suggest that Kam is deprived whilst Karren is very fortunate! Karren has her mother's company all day! Thinking about it in more detail, it becomes obvious that the quality of care may be at least as important as the quantity of care. Kam has other adults to build attachments to. Is Kam really deprived or is it Karren who is suffering privation?

Privation

Rutter approached the effects of deprivation in separate categories – 'short-term' effects (referring to the immediate response after deprivation), and 'long-term' effects (which can be seen over a number of months or years). He concluded that:

1 Most long-term effects are due to the lack of something – which he termed 'privation'– rather than to any type of loss (deprivation).
2 Failure to develop bonds with anyone (not just the mother) is the main factor in developing Bowlby's 'affectionless psychopathy'.
3 The lack of a stable relationship and family discord are more associated with later delinquency and/or anti-social behaviour.
4 Under-achievement is likely to be caused by lack of stimulation and necessary life experiences.

Rutter sums all this up in his book *Maternal Deprivation Reassessed* (2nd edition, 1981):

Mothering is a rather general term which includes a wide range of activities. Love, the development of enduring bonds, a stable but not necessarily unbroken

> relationship, and a 'stimulating' interaction are all necessary qualities but there are many more. Children also need food, care and protection, discipline, models of behaviour, play and conversation. It seems unlikely that all of these have the same role in a child's psychological development . . . (p. 30).
>
> New research has confirmed that, although an important stress, separation is not the crucial factor in most varieties of deprivation. Investigations have also demonstrated the importance of a child's relationship with people other than his mother. Most important of all there has been the repeated finding that many children are not damaged by deprivation. (p. 217)

Rutter therefore suggests that making assumptions about deprivation and the possibility of emotional and social difficulties and under-achievement needs to be looked at carefully. Children often appear to be extremely resilient within a situation of deprivation and the effects might be offset by changes in their care during their early experience. This view is echoed by Barbara Tizard and Jill Hodges (1978, 1979) who studied differences, in terms of emotional, social and intellectual behaviour, between ex-institutional children and ordinary children. Overall, these studies emphasised the beneficial effects of enrichment (or environmental improvement), even in middle or later childhood, which further shows the possibility and even probability of how resilient children can be.

How does this section of the chapter fit with the overall theme in terms of assumptions we may make about others? We may see television programmes or other media reports about crime being related to broken homes and single parents. What has been shown by Rutter, Tizard and Hodges and others is that these assumptions need to be challenged at least, and perhaps done away with altogether, particularly in certain individual situations where any effects of deprivation have been cancelled out by later enrichments in the lives of the children concerned.

Piaget's theory of cognitive development

Childhood learning was a key area for Bowlby and Rutter. Another theorist in the area of child development, Jean Piaget, has been historically influential in our understanding of cognitive development or thinking development.

Piaget theorised that the cognitive development of children was different to that of adults in a number of ways, i.e. the thinking capacity of a child of seven was not simply a 'watered-down' or less well-informed version of an adult's thinking capacity. Piaget believed that children understood the world in a different way to adults.

Piaget's methods of collecting evidence to support his theory have been criticised, as have his methods of research. He used methods of 'naturalistic observation' and the 'clinical interview'. This means he observed children's activities in detail, talked to them and listened to them talking to each other. He also devised and presented 'tests' of ability on this basis. There was none of the manipulation of variables that you might find in most experimental research. Piaget was not interested in the uniqueness of individual children but in the similarities of children's abilities at an equivalent age, say seven to eleven.

Piaget's developmental stages are:

1 Sensori-motor (birth to 2 years approximately)
2 Pre-operational (2–7 years approximately)

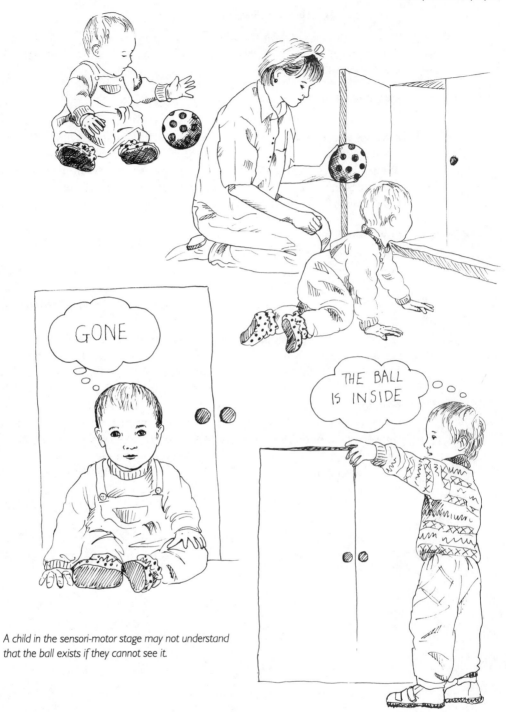

A child in the sensori-motor stage may not understand
that the ball exists if they cannot see it.

At the pre-operational stage the child can imagine the
ball and understand where to find it.

3 Concrete operations (7–11 years approximately)

4 Formal operations (approximately 11 years onwards).

It is important to look at each stage individually in terms of the cognitive development that Piaget's theories would expect to take place.

Stage 1 – Sensori-motor

The young infant's experience of the world during this stage occurs mainly through physical activities and immediate perceptions, as memory, language and therefore 'adult thinking', are not available to the child. The 'permanence' of objects occurs at about eight months (approximately), when children realise that a previously visible object (e.g. a ball) still exists in the toy cupboard even though it is not in front of them in the 'here and now'. Towards the end of this stage, children attain concepts of the future and the past.

Stage 2 – Pre-operational

This stage was of the most interest to Piaget as it involves a long period of basic mental building and development, laying the foundation for operational thinking attained at around age seven, depending on each child's genetically influenced maturation. The key features of the pre-operational stage are what Piaget termed 'egocentrism' and 'centration'.

Egocentrism means that a child can't see things from any other point of view but his or her own. For example, if a child is asked what someone can see from across the road, the scene will be described from their own point of view. Similarly, a little boy may tell you that he has a brother, but he won't usually be able to accept that his brother has a brother!

Piaget's famous 'three mountains task' supposedly illustrated this. Children were shown a picture of three mountains viewed firstly from the front and secondly from the top and asked to select the 'top' view that corresponded to the 'front' view already seen from a selection of photographs. Piaget found that children under eight were unable to imagine what another view of the same mountains would be like.

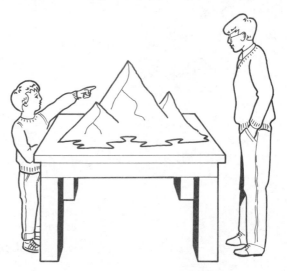

If an egocentric child looked at a model of mountains they would imagine that another person would see the mountains exactly as they saw them. The child would not understand that things look different from different view points.

Centration was tested by Piaget's famous conservation experiments. In these, children were presented with two things the same, i.e. two pieces of plasticine, two beakers of water, two rows of counters, and then one of them was altered in front of the children and they were asked if they were still the same in amount. So the two fat beakers of liquid were shown to the child and then the contents of one was poured into a tall, thin beaker. The child supposedly should say that there is more liquid in the tall, thin beaker than in the fat beaker.

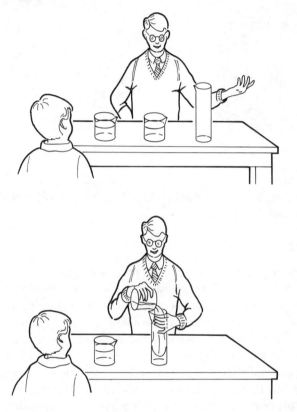

The child will agree that there is the same water in each of the fat beakers, yet when the water is poured into the tall beaker, the child may say that there is now more water in the tall beaker!

Piaget also believed that children's inability to decentre (take all things in a situation into account, not centring on one) was linked to their inability to reverse their thinking. That is, reversibility is used when we realise that $2 \times 3 = 6$, and equally $6/3 = 2$, mentally going back to the starting point.

When children have achieved decentring and operational thinking, they will have attained Stage 3 – Concrete operations.

Stage 3 – Concrete operations

Piaget maintained that conservation in Stage 3 happened in a definitive order, number first and volume last, at about eleven or twelve years of age. This stage was called concrete operations because children need real objects to experiment with in order to solve problems logically. For example, children at this stage may have difficulty in working out the verbal problem, 'Yasmin is taller than Sarah, Yasmin is smaller than

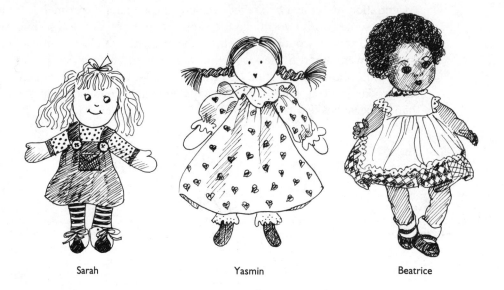

Sarah   Yasmin   Beatrice

Beatrice, who is the smallest?', but no difficulty if given three dolls to represent Yasmin, Sarah and Beatrice.

Stage 4 – Formal operations

This stage is marked by the ability to see things in an abstract sense, without the need for concrete or visual representation. Children's thinking here increasingly becomes more like an adult's. Problems can be solved in their heads; children can test out different ideas, see them separately and also how they link together. Formal operational thinking takes many years to achieve and not everyone necessarily achieves it. Further, Piaget's theories are typically 'eurocentric': that is, based on Western scientists' concept of formal logic. Some societies have other forms of logic that may differ, but are still used to reason logically through culturally specific problems, different to those used by Piaget.

As mentioned before, Piaget's importance in psychology is largely historical. His contributions to education, particularly at the primary school level, have been huge; children are no longer viewed as passive beings shaped by their environment. Because of Piaget's work, children started to be seen as active seekers of knowledge learning by 'discovery'. Despite this very real contribution Piaget has had many critics. For example, McGarrigle and Donaldson (1978), along with Hughes (1975), criticise Piaget's methods as being unfair to young children. Donaldson has shown that very young children (between three and a half and five) are not necessarily egocentric if the tasks are presented in different ways. Children can conserve number as Donaldson's 'naughty teddy' experiment showed. The 'naughty teddy' moved the row of counters and turned the experiment into more of a game. Children were able to conserve number and report that the counters were the same when the situation was personalised and fun.

Margaret Donaldson in her book *Children's Minds* (1978) states:

> . . . pre-school children are not nearly so limited in their ability to 'decentre', or appreciate someone else's point of view, as Piaget has for many years maintained . . . The abandonment of belief in pronounced childhood egocentrism has far-reaching

> implications. But its significance will be better understood if it is seen in the light of recent evidence and arguments about the ways in which children learn to use and understand language. (p. 30)

Margaret Donaldson mentions new thinking about cognition such as metacognition. Her work puts Piaget's contribution firmly within a historical context.

Understanding our thinking – are 'formal operations' really a stage of development?

Piaget's view of intellectual development suggests that the great achievement of adults is that they develop formal logical reasoning. The child or adolescent may think in terms of concrete logical operations. This limits what the adolescent can understand. Practical examples can be remembered but abstract concepts and abstract reasoning may be too difficult. Piaget's stage of formal operations or 'formal logical operations' suggested that most adults could cope with abstract concepts because they were more logical.

This focus on logic is criticised by David Cohen (1983). Cohen pointed out that being able to use formal deductive logic is a useful skill; it may have seemed the peak of human achievement in the 1930s. Nowadays, many adults may not need formal logic very often. Formal logic is a specialised way of thinking invented by the ancient Greeks. It can be useful for solving certain kinds of puzzles and is central to mathematical and some philosophical problem solving. A study by Johnstone-Laird in 1972 found that many university students were not able to use formal operations to solve logical puzzles. Cohen also quotes studies in the USA which suggest that there is no 'natural' developmental sequence involving formal logical ability.

Since the 1970s, many psychologists have become interested in an alternative to Formal Operations. What may distinguish the expert care manager from a younger person may not really be their use of logic. Instead, it may be that adults learn to monitor their own thinking. Adults may learn skills in evaluating ideas and using concepts to remember things. Younger people may not have developed this ability to its full potential. The expert care manager may be able to hold a conversation with a client. While the client is talking, the care manager will not only listen, but will also think through useful concepts which might explain what the client is saying. Perhaps the client is an elder, and perhaps they are talking about loneliness and how things used to be better. The care manager can use concepts like depression, disempowerment, helplessness, threat to self-esteem and identity in order to understand the situation. Not only this, but the care manager can analyse their own thoughts, they can think: 'Why am I thinking this person is depressed – perhaps this is a wrong assumption – I could check it out by asking a question here.'

The ability to analyse your own ideas or thoughts is a special kind of thinking or cognitive skill. Flavell (1979) calls this skill 'metacognition'. 'Meta' means 'beyond' or 'higher level', so 'metacognition' means beyond ordinary thinking, or it can mean higher level thinking. Metacognition is the ability to understand, monitor and evaluate your own thoughts. Because metacognition involves understanding and controlling personal thoughts, it is often called metacognitive knowledge. You have knowledge of how your own thought processes work!

So, an expert carer may be able to understand and assess clients' needs not only because they listen, not only because they know a lot of theory, not only because they have lots of experience, but perhaps mostly because they understand their own thinking!

Flavell (1979) believed that the ability to understand and control personal thinking processes might lead on to metacognitive experiences. These experiences might involve more self-control and confidence. It may be that the ability to think about your own thoughts and understand them leads to greater understanding of other people. If you can question your own thinking while talking to a client, then you can adjust your ideas and questions to that client as you go along. The ability to question or monitor your own thoughts may involve metacognition. If you know you are good at this, you may feel confident about your skills, you might also feel more confident about your whole ability to assess and understand yourself and others.

Reflective activity

Think of a client you have met and worked with. What words or concepts might you use to describe this person? Maybe you would like to make a note of these words. Now ask yourself why you chose these concepts. How accurate are these ideas really? Would there be any other ways of describing the person? Can you imagine your own 'self' asking 'you' these questions? If you can imagine yourself asking 'you' questions and you can answer these questions, then you are monitoring your own thinking. Develop this as a skill and you are developing metacognitive knowledge.

Metacognition may be a kind of reasoning skill, but it is not the same as thinking logically. Metacognition may be far more important than formal logical operations when it comes to skilled understanding of other people, assessment and decision making. It may be that adult experts are different from more 'concrete' workers because they understand their own thinking.

As David Cohen, in his book *Piaget – Critique and Reassessment* (1983), states:

> It is certainly true that part of Piaget's work has not dated. It is also true that his semi-naturalistic approach to observations has much to offer today's psychology. It would be nice to have observations which were actually more naturalistic and more rounded than his – including the child's social and family life – while also ensuring that some of the methodologies used were more rigorous . . . His concern to have the infant move through one stage after another; his ignoring of social, class and individual differences; his hankering after a universal theory of human growth – all mark him out as a past master rather than a contemporary one . . . He deserves to be honoured and remembered as one of the great psychologists, but as a psychologist of the past. Developmental psychology has started to move in quite different directions – and needs to. (p. 152)

Evidence opportunity

Talk to a young child, an older child and an adult. Ask them about their friends and how they get on at school or at work. Not only will each person have very different experiences to describe, but their way of understanding life is likely to be different. Try to use concepts of stages of development to explain some of the differences you discover.

Personality

Cross-cultural considerations need to be looked at to gain a wider appreciation of many of the theories and ideas we have come across so far in this chapter. Theories like Erikson's psycho-social development (see Chapter 2) may do this quite well. Others like Freud's, Bowlby's and Piaget's theories do this less well. The torchlight metaphor may be useful here to view different theories and how they each might relate to the assumptions we may make about others. What about the concept of personality and situational influences in perceiving other people?

There are different perspectives in psychology such as psychodynamic, behaviourist, cognitive, humanistic and neurobiological. Each perspective has a corresponding view of personality and a view of mental health and treatment for mental illness. For example, Freud and Erikson provide views of personality in the psychodynamic tradition, Skinner in the behaviourist tradition.

The neurobiological perspective explains personality as being dependent on the brain, as Hans Eysenck (1965) theorised. Eysenck's theory of personality is also known as a 'type' theory of personality.

Eysenck used human physiology as a basis for explaining the enduring features of each individual that we refer to as personality. The assumption is that biology provides a foundation or starting point for explaining personality. Eysenck developed one of the most appealing theories of personality based on such a set of assumptions.

Eysenck traced his theory back to the ancient Greek physician (or doctor), Galen (129–199 AD). Galen had tried to understand human behaviour in relation to a theory of humours or temperaments. This theory stated that each person was influenced by a balance of four body fluids: blood, phlegm, black bile, and yellow bile.

- Blood created a 'sanguine' base for a person's temperament; it caused a cheerful and active disposition.
- Phlegm created a phlegmatic temperament which was supposed to be calm and apathetic.
- Black bile encouraged a melancholic temperament which can be sad and pessimistic.
- Yellow bile caused a choleric temperament which was supposed to be irritable, excitable and aggressive.

Naturally, medicine has long abandoned this belief in fluids influencing people in such a way. Eysenck argued that whilst the location of the cause was incorrect, Galen's observations of human temperament were right.

People's general way of reacting to life might fit a set of descriptions as shown on p. 78.

Eysenck's basic theory is that an area of the human mid-brain called the 'reticular formation' can work in different ways in different individuals. The reticular formation is believed to have an influence on how alert or 'aroused' an individual is in relation to the events around them.

In simplified form, Eysenck hypothesises (theorises) that in some people the reticular formation has a tendency to 'overplay' signals from the outside world and create a high level of arousal to events which are not really very important. In other people, the reticular formation is 'sluggish' and doesn't get the whole central nervous system excited unless very strong messages are coming in from outside. So while a person may see or hear certain messages, they won't really react and take notice unless the reticular formation 'boosts the signal' so that the message creates an impact. People with very active reticular formations are introverts, according to Eysenck, and people with very sluggish systems are extroverts.

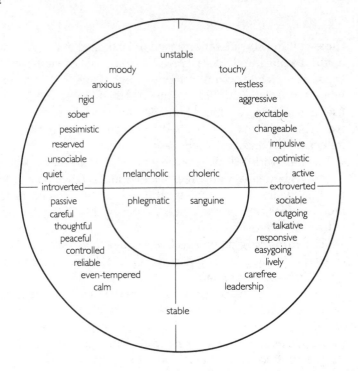

Eysenck's theory of introversion and extroversion, unstable and stable personality types. Taken from Fact and Fiction in Psychology *(1965) p. 54. Galen's four temperaments are described in the centre.*

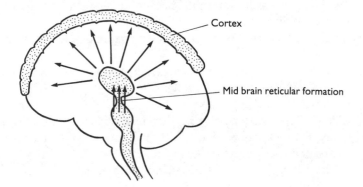

Inside the brain – the reticular formation

Eysenck has taken these terms from a theory of Carl Jung who had previously used them to indicate a disposition to inner or outward exploration of the self. In Eysenck's theory, an introvert is a person with a nervous system that can become easily overstimulated. An extrovert is an individual whose nervous system is potentially difficult to arouse. So the extrovert is stimulus hungry; desperate for experience and excitement in order to function properly at a fully operational mental level. Most people are hypothesised to be neither extreme introverts or extreme extroverts, but somewhere in between these two 'type' descriptions, i.e. average!

Eysenck adds the dimension of unstable (or neurotic) versus stable to describe an emotional dimension which interacts with introversion/extroversion. Eysenck believes that this dimension is based on differences in an individual's nervous system and the limbic system of the mid-brain which controls it. These biological systems in turn influence how a person learns and experiences their life. Specifically, Eysenck claims that introverts will be more responsive to conditioned learning than will extroverts. Introverts will learn more quickly and with fewer experiences to create associations. Because introverts react more strongly to conditioning, introversion may influence their personality or personality traits. Finally, many other influences exist which can affect behaviour, but Eysenck believes that the tendency to condition will influence not only an individual's disposition, but also their real-life behaviour. In his 1966 work *Fact and Fiction in Psychology*, Eysenck did claim to have evidence that criminal behaviour was more associated with extroverted and unstable test scores than with other test results.

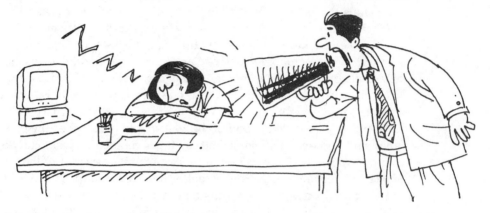

Extroverts are thought to need a lot of 'stimulation' and excitement to enable them to function properly!

The theory creates a very impressive explanation for the biological basis of behaviour and for the importance of biological temperament (in this instance based on conditioned learning and emotional reaction). However, there are problems with the theory – it is not necessarily accepted as being true (see Mark Cook, 1984).

The first problem is that the reticular formation and the limbic system have not been proved to act in the way that Eysenck suggests they do.

Secondly, the evidence for conditioned learning really being linked to traits that can be measured by tests is contested (argued about between different researchers).

Mark Cook (1984) also questions whether the methodology and foundations of the theory are as sound and secure as they seem at first.

From a care perspective, we also have to question the usefulness of the theory. It may be useful to think about a biological core or temperament at the heart of personality; people may be influenced by biology as well as by learning, perception and social context. If some people are hungry for stimulation, and others are keen to avoid it, this is another aspect of individuality which requires to be valued and respected. The test of usefulness may come down to: 'can you usefully predict anything more with this theory?'

Perception of others

Trait theories contrast with 'type' theories of personality, such as Eysenck's. The most prominent trait theory is that of Raymond Cattell. Cattell's personality inventory, called the 16PF (PF = personality factors), along with Eysenck's E.P.I. (Eysenck Personality Inventory) originally formed the basis of research questionnaires for investigating personality. They both fall into the 'nomothetic' category of personality theory, that is, they both believe that the behaviour of individuals reflects a relatively enduring personality, and that people can be grouped in terms of types or similarity of traits. Other personality theories see personality as being much more individual and this category is called 'idiographic'. Personality can also be seen as situational or strongly influenced by context (Mischel, 1965). Cattell, however, saw personality as 'what determines behaviour in a defined situation and a defined mood' (Cattell, 1965).

Another trait theory and a more traditional one is that of Soloman Asch. This is a theory of implicit personality, which distinguishes between descriptive traits and evaluative traits. That is, knowing whether someone is honest or deceitful, trustworthy or treacherous, likeable or unlikeable (evaluative) is more central to us than knowing whether someone is blonde or brunette, tall or short (descriptive).

Asch conducted an experiment with some students involving two lists of personality traits which were suppose to describe an external speaker due to visit. Both lists had the same traits on them, for example, 'intelligent, skilful, industrious, warm, determined, practical, cautious', except that 'warm' was replaced by 'cold' on the second list. Each student was given only one list and was asked to rate the external speaker afterwards.

As Asch expected, 90 per cent of the 'warm' group described the person as 'generous, happy and good-natured' compared to 10 per cent, 35 per cent and 25 per cent of the 'cold' group for those three characteristics. Sixty-five per cent of the 'warm' group said he was 'wise' compared to 30 per cent of the 'cold' group. The 'cold' group evaluated him as 'mean, unfriendly, miserable, humourless and unliked'. Both groups showed what Asch had predicted: 'warm' and 'cold' are 'central' traits; other less important ones are called 'peripheral', e.g. punctuality, tiredness, etc.

The above study explains implicit personality theory (the central traits cause 'other' traits that you could feel might be in character for either a 'warm' or a 'cold' person). The study also involves what is known as the 'primacy effect'.

Primacy and recency

A famous study described by Asch in the 1940s, was developed by Kelley (1950) and Wishner (1960) with comparable results. Implicit personality theory is clearly important, along with the 'primacy–recency' effect (Luchins, 1957). Impression formation is the interactive process, in which we form impressions of others. These impressions can, and do, often change over time as the person or people concerned become better known to you. However, the belief in first impressions being extremely important, and perhaps even crucial, as for example in job interviews, is a view that is widely held.

The primacy–recency effect also shows this. Primacy involves 'priming' people with information in advance. To use the 'job interview' scenario, this would perhaps be the way you put yourself across on the application form. 'Recency' is seen to be just as important in some situations, particularly legal ones, which is perhaps why the case for the defence is usually put last to the jury before they decide the verdict or outcome of the trial.

Information that is received immediately before making a judgement of any kind is more likely to be retained and used than information given, say, two days before that.

Luchins' (1957) study involved two paragraphs of information about a boy called Jim, and students were asked to rate Jim on the basis of what they had been primed with or told. Both groups of students were read the 'extrovert' paragraph (a) and the 'introvert' paragraph (b).

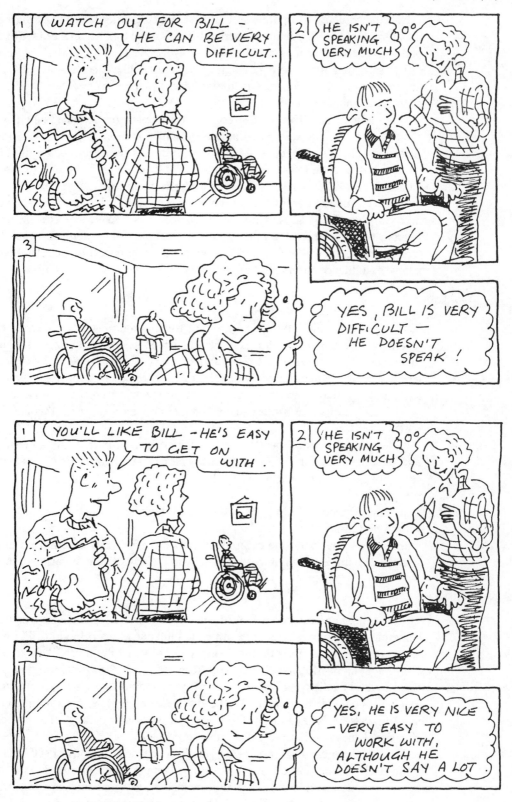

Primacy – the power of suggestion

Half the students had paragraph (a) first, and the other half had paragraph (b) first. Of the (a)-first group, 52 per cent described Jim as an extrovert, and of the (b)-first group, 56 per cent described him as an introvert. Only 12 per cent (a), and 10 per cent (b), respectively, said that they were not sure. This study, like Asch's and Kelley's, shows the importance of these processes in interpersonal perception and how easily we can make assumptions about others.

There is evidence that we use cognitive processes or 'schema' when we try to learn about others. A schema is past knowledge which is used to interpret current experience. A schema (plural schemata) will help us with the overwhelming amount of information in all the social situations we encounter. We use these 'schema' to 'infer', or make judgements either in terms of personality traits, as in implicit personality, or on the basis of given information as in the 'primacy–recency' effect. Inference is a cognitive process, involving our thinking, and just as we sometimes perceive objects, in an almost fixed fashion, we might perceive other people in this way too. Inference is involved in stereotyping. Stereotypes allow past assumptions about physical or occupational attributes of people to influence our interaction with them.

Stereotypes

Stereotypes generally only have a grain of truth to them, and people may try hard not to 'live up to the stereotype', for example, the schoolteacher who dresses casually and likes to be called by their first name. Stereotypes can be 'self-fulfilling'; for example, if you were labelled as being 'aggressive', you might find that others interpreted your behaviour as such, and you may even start behaving aggressively. Stereotypes can also be long-lasting as in the case of gender-roles; many women and men can find this an almost constant obstacle in their lives.

Our attitudes to other people can usually consist, in part, of stereotypes, and they can also be long-lasting and very difficult to change. The reason for this is because attitudes consist of three component parts:

- cognitive
- affective (involving feelings and deeply held beliefs)
- behavioural.

Studies show that only one component part can effectively be changed at any one time, nevertheless this is heavily targeted socially in the advertising of various products.

Attribution

The other area of inference is that of 'attribution' where we attribute a cause or reason for something happening, usually in terms of someone else's behaviour. For example, if you see someone with a smile on their face, you are generally more likely to attribute this to their being a cheerful, capable person, rather than to their situation being happy at that time. Even skilled psychologists (who perhaps should know better!) can make what Fritz Heider called the 'fundamental attribution error', that is, assuming that the cause of someone else's behaviour is the result of personal factors like mood, rather than situational ones which can often be more important.

The fundamental attribution error can also occur in situations of self-attribution. We are more likely to interpret our own success as being a result of our skill or competence – if others are successful, we are usually inclined to say that they are just lucky! There are several sources of bias in attribution which contribute to these errors.

Self-concept

Our self-concept is obviously key here; if we have high self-esteem the above situation is more likely to occur than not. The other parts of self-concept are self-image and 'ideal self'. This was mentioned in the previous chapters, particularly in relation to Cooley's 'looking-glass self' and the theories of Carl Rogers.

Rogers' concept of ideal self suggests great potential in being human, that we are capable of great love and tolerance of one another, and that this love can heal us in situations of difficulty or states of what he called 'incongruence'. Like Abraham Maslow, his fellow humanistic theorist, Rogers sees almost a 'drive' towards becoming 'congruent' or whole, achievement of the ideal self being possible for everyone through his 'client-centred' therapy, where people were given 'unconditional positive regard'.

Maslow, however, sees his 'self-actualisation' as being achievable by very few – his basic theory was also discussed in Chapter 2. He did nevertheless see his 'hierarchy of needs' (see diagram on p. 51) as being central to all human experience.

Social influences

Michael Argyle, in his book *The Psychology of Interpersonal Behaviour* (1983, reprinted 1990), sees human behaviour in social situations as purposeful, goal directed, and motivationally driven. He states: 'Different people seek different things in social situations' (p. 11).

> In the present state of knowledge it looks as if social behaviour is the product of different drives. A 'drive' can be defined as a persistent tendency to seek certain goals. Besides directing people towards goals, a drive is a source of energy; when the drive is operating there is a general increase of vigour. Much the same is true of biological drives, such as the need for food: when a person is hungry they will seek food with increased effort.
>
> Biological drives can be sub-divided into a number of more specific ones for salt, sugar and so on: animals deprived of one of these substances may select a diet which makes good the deficit. It is necessary to theorise these various forms of motivation to account for variations in the behaviour of the *same* person on different occasions, e.g. when hungry and not, and to describe differences between *different* people in the goals they pursue, and the energy with which they do it. There is as yet no final agreement on how social motivation should be divided up.

On a previous page in his book, Argyle proposes social skills training as being essential in social interaction. Training which, ultimately, would eradicate some of the problems and also some of the assumptions that we make about others.

> Many people are lonely and unhappy, some are mentally ill, because they are unable to establish and sustain social relationships with others. Many everyday encounters are unpleasant, embarrassing or fruitless, because of inept social behaviour. Conflicts between different social classes and different cultural groups are partly due to the difficulties of interaction. Many of those difficulties and frustrations could be

eliminated by a wider understanding, and better training in the skills of social interaction. (p. 9)

Drive theory, as social motivation, effectively explains human behaviour in many situations: the 'drive to succeed', for example, or in the social learning context, the drive to imitate and learn social behaviour.

Albert Bandura stressed the importance of observational learning and modelling. In his famous 'bo-bo doll' experiment, he showed how children effectively learn to be aggressive by observing and modelling adult behaviour. The experiment involved children watching violent television programmes and then observing different adults beating up an inflatable doll in another room. Bandura's results showed that most of the children imitated the adults and behaved aggressively, so the influence of the violent programme as a 'primer' can't be ruled out. The extent of observational learning and modelling adopted by children after viewing 'video nasties' cannot be adequately monitored.

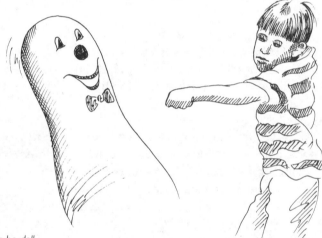

Child hitting the bo-bo doll

Assumptions can often be, and usually are, something of a limitation in trying to understand other people. Like the other material covered so far in this book, it is as well to point out that we need to be aware that we are only obtaining 'clues' – partial illumination, to use the torch metaphor – and that none of the theories available will give us absolute knowledge about others, no matter how interesting or influential they are. The reason for this is that human beings are undeniably individual, unique and multi-faceted, and psychology reveals this each time it tries to explore human behaviour scientifically.

There are always going to be fundamental problems with trying to understand people; however, with each new study that pushes the boundaries of our current understanding, we can't help but find our curiosity aroused by the fascination of trying to find out about the complexities of what makes us human.

Whether ideas come from the psychodynamic, behaviourist, neurobiological, cognitive, humanistic, or social learning perspective, we may gain the clearest picture and the most illumination if we take all the ideas together. By superimposing them one on the other, if at all possible, we can lay the foundations for psychological understanding within the context of health and social care.

Evidence opportunity

Observe a situation in a care setting where you or other care workers try to provide individualised care. Talk to the workers or reflect on your own work. Ask yourself or the others how they see the needs of the individuals they are working with. Can you find processes of attribution, social influence, primacy, stereotyping or other perceptual issues at work?

4 Coping with strong emotions

What is covered in this chapter

- Aggression in caring contexts
- Context and threat
- Making sense of aggression
- Coping with stress
- Stress management techniques

Reflective activity

Think of any recent experiences you have had of visiting a hospital, an out-patient department, a rest home or a day centre for elders.

- How many people did you notice who were in pain, how many were unhappy?
- Were some individuals threatened by loneliness, by a fear of being socially devalued?
- Was anyone worried, frustrated, impatient?
- Were any of the people you met afraid – fearful of what might happen to them, or what illnesses they might have?
- Have you seen relatives who are worried or upset for their children, or indeed, their parents?

Aggression in caring contexts

Health and Social Care work often involves working with kind, generous and grateful clients. It would be wrong to build an image of constantly working with stressed, difficult or angry people. But, thinking about the care situations above, there must be many individuals who are experiencing very emotionally charged situations. Sometimes these situations may create anger, verbal abuse or outright aggression and violence.

Glynis Breakwell (1989) quotes a study in 1986 by the Health and Safety Commission into violence in the Health Service. The study revealed that: 'one in 200 workers had suffered a major injury following a violent attack during the preceding year. A further one in 10 needed first aid and one in 20 had been threatened with knives, chairs, broken bottles, and the like. As many as one in six had been threatened verbally' (Breakwell, 1989, p. 29).

Breakwell goes on to suggest: 'If these official figures are taken seriously, it seems that Health Service workers are at least 26 times more likely to be seriously injured than the general public' (Breakwell, 1989, p. 29). In the Social Services, a national survey showed one assault for every 259 posts on average per year (Breakwell, 1989, p. 32).

More recently, studies in one London borough (1990 to 1992) recorded that approximately 27 per cent of all recorded accidents in Social Services were in fact assaults. Again, about 46 per cent of all accidents reported by care assistants were assaults. Yet, as Glynis Breakwell observes: 'It is strange how few members of the caring professions are ever trained directly to handle powerful emotions . . . practitioners have minimal instruction on how to deal with these emotions' (Breakwell, 1989, p. 17).

The risk of aggression, and the need to know what to do in order to cope, are vital areas for study in Health and Social Care. Practical coping will depend on experience – the careworker's own experience, and other people's! In addition to experience, concepts and theory can guide a worker's reactions. Theory works because it can enable a person to understand a situation. If we can understand then we can predict what to expect; if we know what to expect we may be able to feel in control of our own emotions. Theory can also increase personal confidence by enabling people to analyse and evaluate what has happened in the past. Without theory we have to invent our own personal explanations for aggression. Without any explanations, aggression can leave a person anxious, fearful and unable to know what to expect.

Alternatively, the easy way of responding to aggression by 'fighting back' requires no theory. One problem with 'fighting back' is that it is unacceptable in a care setting, where the careworker is required to work within a value base.

Knowing how to cope with aggression or abuse will also involve knowing how to cope with our own thoughts.

Context and threat

Reflective activity

Imagine yourself starting a new job in care and you have been working for just a few days; perhaps working with children, perhaps working with people with learning disabilities, perhaps with elders.

- **Working with children**: You have been organising a play session and are now encouraging the children to put away their toys. One child throws a toy at you and shouts: 'I hate you.' Other staff look up and stare at you.
- **Working with people with learning disabilities**: You are walking down the corridor talking to a colleague when one of the members of the centre spits at you.
- **Working with elders**: You are helping an older woman to put her shoes on, you are kneeling down, when suddenly you are slapped in the face by the woman's hand. Nothing was said, there was no warning!

In all the above situations the physical damage is very limited. The toy will bounce off your body with no effects. The spit contains no risky substances and can soon be wiped off. The slap may leave a slight, temporary mark, but it goes away within 20 minutes. It is not the physical risk that is threatening in these situations. These situations might cause threat to a worker's self-esteem, their self-concept or identity.

Feelings of anger, fear, or loss of confidence, might follow an assault. Feelings of guilt or helplessness might even result from being attacked by a client. The impact of an assault will depend on the social meaning that is placed on the incident. Imagine the difference between the following contexts:

Having a toy thrown at you

- Context 1: You are working with a young child who has learned to get their own way by having temper tantrums. The staff all understand this and are trying to provide attention when the child is not aggressive. Aggressive behaviour is confronted gently but firmly, by telling the child to stop. The staff look at you expecting you to follow an agreed care plan approach.
- Context 2: The child usually gets on with all the other staff, and children. The way the staff look at you suggests that they think you have done something wrong. A senior member of staff asks if they can have a word with you outside.

In the first situation the child's anger is expected. A skilled careworker might immediately think about the child's care plan and how they need to be careful not to reinforce the child's aggression (see p. 43). The careworker has the support of their colleagues. There is no attack on the carer's self-concept.

In the second situation the carer might have cause to feel upset. It looks as if the other staff see the aggression as the carer's fault. The carer might feel incompetent, not able to control the situation. The carer might feel angry, or afraid that they don't understand the situation. Upsetting a young child might be a cause for guilt.

Being spat at

Again, there is a world of difference between a colleague who knows the client and can explain the behaviour to you, and a colleague who looks shocked and says: 'I wonder why the member did that to you.' Being spat at is quite an intense insult or form of abuse. If we feel that the way we look, the way we act, the gender or race that we represent is the reason for the attack, then our own identity or self-concept may be threatened. If we understand why the client behaves this way, we may be less threatened. Support from colleagues is important to help us protect our own identity.

Being slapped

This always hurts! Once the initial shock passes, it is the social meaning which may create a lasting threat. If the resident hit out in pain or because they were disorientated, it doesn't make it alright, but it does enable us to understand the situation. If we can understand what was happening we may be able to prevent it from happening again.

If a carer can understand, and predict what may happen, then there is no need for fear or anxiety when working with the client. If hitting is just purely random, purely out of control and unpredictable, then it may be impossible to carry on caring. Naturally any assault, spitting or hitting is a serious attack and it should always be reported and recorded.

In order to feel that it is possible to cope with aggression, a person must be able to make sense of the aggression. Making sense of aggression may require a knowledge of the client, a knowledge of the client's situation, an awareness of own self-concept, and a range of concepts and theories for understanding aggression.

Making sense of aggression

The great difficulty with aggression is that it can make a careworker feel threatened. Threat can cause fear. Threat may be associated with not being able to predict or guess how we will behave or how another person will behave. If we did know what to expect from ourselves or others then we might feel safer. Sometimes, just believing that we know what to expect may be enough to make a person feel safe or in control. Theory can be really useful – not because it always works – but just because it provides an explanation.

If a careworker believes that they can understand what is happening, the belief itself can create a sense of safety. If we feel safe we may communicate more clearly. If we feel in control we may have the confidence to cope with difficult situations. Believing that you understand what will happen may be enough to enable you to cope. Theory may turn out to be a practical tool for carers to use. Sometimes it will work because the confidence it gives will cause things to turn out alright. Theory doesn't have to be one hundred per cent correct for it to work!

Chapter 2 featured the situation where an older man became abusive when a careworker took him a cup of tea. Very often aggression and abuse happen suddenly or at least they seem to happen suddenly. Usually there is no time to start to reflect and theorise. Because of this it is easy to lose control of the situation. Typically the client might have been feeling angry about his life. Perhaps no one has talked to him for several hours. Perhaps he feels neglected.

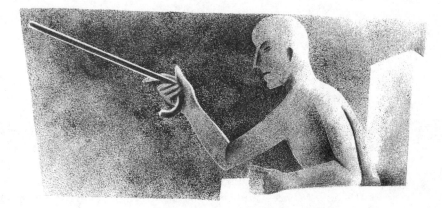

While he is sitting he begins to look tense. Perhaps the man will squeeze both hands together, stare at the floor, tense his face and jaw. The careworker is busy, the client looks tense, but the careworker hopes that they will just have a short chat and then they can get on with other things. The careworker offers the tea but doesn't acknowledge the client's tension. Instead, they say something about being in a hurry. The man is in a private reality of pain and tension, while the careworker is in another private world of 'being busy'. Next, the client explodes with anger. His needs have not been acknowledged or met so he abuses the careworker. This causes the careworker to feel threatened and angry. The careworker backs away but they resent the client's behaviour. Their own self-concept is threatened. The careworker may want to get back at the client. They may feel a need to 'get their own back', how dare anyone treat them like this!

Question: How can theory help in this situation?

Answer: It can't! Theory is only useful if it has been learned before and if it guides the way the careworker thinks about their situation.

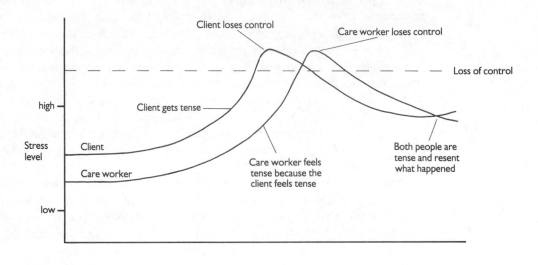

Client and careworker stress levels

The problem is that the client's stress has caused the careworker to become stressed. Both client and careworker may be in danger of losing control.

The careworker might have been able to stay in control by using a selection of techniques which create self-confidence. These include:

- Using work role theory to protect self-concept and self-confidence.
- Using conditioned learning to practise and learn to control personal, emotional responses.
- Using assertive behaviour.
- Using self-concept and other cognitive techniques to control emotion.
- Using calming and conversational skills as appropriate to the social context.
- Using theory as a defence mechanism.

Using 'work role' theory

The careworker could immediately think of the situation in terms of social role. The abuse is being directed at him or her as a careworker. The abuse isn't necessarily directed at personal self-concept or identity. Verbal abuse may not shock the careworker if they feel that their role at work includes overhearing such things. The abuse may not be taken personally if the careworker's social role acts as a buffer between the client's behaviour and the worker's identity or self-concept. The careworker can think things like: 'OK, this is one of the things that happen here – as a careworker I can cope, I'll stay calm and try and sort it out.'

For this kind of thought process to work, the careworker would need to have thought about their work role beforehand. They might also need to have thought about the boundaries of their role. Boundaries explain what the careworker is prepared to put up with. The worker may tolerate some kinds of anger but not other kinds. By thinking through the boundaries in advance, the careworker is more likely to stay in control of their own emotions when confronted with abuse. They will know when to withdraw, and

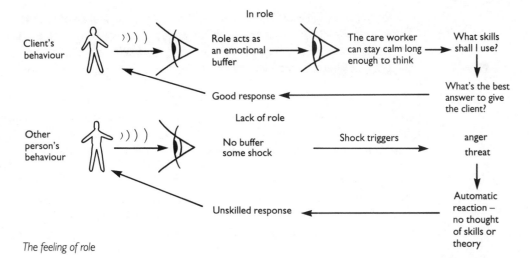

The feeling of role

when to make a formal complaint. Thinking this through in advance should help a careworker to feel confident.

Using conditioned learning theory to control own responses

There is a natural tendency to want to fight or run away if a person feels threatened. This tendency can sometimes be controlled by learning relaxation techniques. Relaxation techniques based on breathing and muscle tension have been used for many centuries by individuals who have practised yoga.

Relaxation is a skill rather than a use of theory, but the idea of conditioned relaxation is an interesting development which uses the behaviourist perspective. The main idea is that an individual learns to tell the difference between tense feelings and relaxed feelings. By identifying tension and relaxation the person can choose to feel relaxed when they need to. The conditioning comes in because the individual learns to associate a word – perhaps the word 'relax' – to the feelings of muscle relaxation.

The best way to learn this is to go for training with an instructor; but here is a basic 'do it yourself' exercise which may explain the idea of learning to control tension through muscle relaxation.

1 Breathe in deeply and tense the muscles in your face, neck, arms, hands and chest. Try to concentrate on what this tension feels like.
2 When the tension is just becoming unpleasant – think 'relax' to yourself. Breathe out slowly through the nose; as you breathe out relax all the areas that were tense. Check that the jaw, the forehead, the neck and the shoulders are limp and free from tension. Try to concentrate on the feeling of calm and relaxation in your muscles.
3 When you have finished breathing out, breathe in fully and tense all your muscles again as before – try to learn what tension feels like.
4 Again, think the word 'relax', breathe out slowly through the nose and check that your face, shoulders, neck and arms are all relaxed. Try to learn the feeling of being relaxed and try to connect the feeling to the word 'relax'.
5 Breathe in again fully – but don't tense your muscles.

6 When you are ready, think 'relax' and try to get the feeling of relaxation fixed in your body – breathe out through the nose slowly concentrating on being relaxed.

7 Repeat stages 5 and 6 again – trying to get the feeling of relaxation and trying to get it connected to the word 'relax'.

This exercise would have to be practised quite a few times in a quiet place where you can be alone and undisturbed. It doesn't work for everyone, you have to be able to believe in it if it is going to have a chance to work. If it does work, what usually happens is that you connect the word 'relax' with a feeling of being relaxed. This means that when you are tense, even thinking of the word 'relax' will remind you of the sensation of being relaxed – you will relax from the tension!

Naturally, this technique needs to be practised many times before the skill of muscle relaxation is learnt. Learning to control personal tension may be like the skill involved in learning to swim. Conditioning feelings of relaxation to a word like 'relax' also takes time to learn. If the conditioned association is built up then all a person has to do is to think 'relax' and relaxed feelings can automatically happen. This power to control personal emotion might help a careworker to feel confident and safe when working with aggressive clients. Learning to relax might also involve 'incompatible stimuli' when it comes to coping with aggression. Stimuli is the plural of stimulus. A stimulus is something that provokes a reaction in a biological system. The words stimuli and stimulus come from a Latin word *stimulare* meaning to goad or whip or beat someone into action.

The term stimuli is most frequently associated with a behaviourist or neurobiological perspective. In these perspectives people are often viewed as organisms which are 'whipped into action' or made to act because of stimuli or pressures in the environment.

The idea of incompatible stimuli refers to pressures which might cancel each other out. If a person is 'presented' with a learned (perhaps conditioned) stimulus to relax, while they are also 'presented' with a stimulus to behave aggressively, the two incompatible stimuli might cancel each other out. In everyday language: someone insults you (a stimulus to react with aggression) but you can think 'relax' (you have trained yourself to be calm when you hear this word). The two stimuli might cancel each other.

Using assertive behaviour

Assertiveness is often seen as 'sticking up for yourself'; it is that – but it isn't just that!

Sometimes people behave in a weak, submissive or withdrawn way, sometimes people behave in an aggressive, dominant, or destructive way. Assertion is the alternative way of behaving which is in between submission and aggression.

Richard Rakos (1986) quotes research which suggests the existence of a continuum (or continuing line) between non-assertion, assertion and aggression when it comes to analysing individual behaviour. Table 4.1 describes how assertion fits between weak and aggressive behaviour.

For example, a weak or non-assertive way of responding to the abusive resident would be to say something like: 'I'm terribly sorry, I didn't mean to say I was in a hurry. I'll try to be better in future.' An aggressive way of responding might be: 'Don't you talk to me like that – you'll wait your turn just like all the rest. If you don't like the way I work, take yourself somewhere else!' Assertion might involve clarifying the situation: 'I can see you're upset with me, but I don't understand why at the moment – can we talk this through?'

Table 4.1

Weakness	Assertion	Aggression
Acceptance of other person's needs	Acceptance of own and other person's needs	Acceptance of own needs
Concern to 'give way'. Other person's needs most important	Concern to negotiate between own and other's needs	Concern to win. Own needs are most important
Puts self down. Critical of self	Behaves fairly, is objective – says 'I believe' or 'I think' when making statements	Puts other people down. Critical of other people
Gives excuses – apologises a lot, probably doesn't listen. Asks questions to find out what's wanted	Listens – no 'shoulds' or 'oughts' – uses questions clearly and calmly. States one's own thoughts and negotiates with others	Accuses others – doesn't listen to others, mind is already made up. Interrupts, is threatening and demanding. Asks few questions.
Doesn't state 'wants'	States 'wants' clearly but negotiates	States demands not 'wants'

Both weak and aggressive responses fix the worker into a particular way of responding. Assertion provides the worker with a chance to sort things out, while staying in control of personal emotion.

Assertion involves awareness of own and others' needs. Assertive behaviour involves trying to negotiate. It involves being able to stick up for yourself without becoming weak or aggressive.

Non-verbal assertion is likely to involve:

- being calm
- using a steady, firm, normal voice
- being clear in speech
- altering facial expressions as your feelings change
- normal eye contact but 'firm' gaze.

Aggression might involve:

- a loud voice
- speech which is fast and abrupt
- scowls and stares
- tense muscles, angry expressions – closed hands and tense movements.

Being assertive will probably increase confidence in working with people. If we can switch to a chosen way of behaving and feel in control of ourselves, then we have another reason to 'feel good'. Feeling good about ourselves may lead to confidence!

Being assertive is not easy, especially when others are being aggressive or threatening. We may have a desire to run away, or we have a desire to get even – 'Right, I'll hurt you if you're going to hurt me!'

As Richard Rakos (1986) points out, assertion is not a personality trait. Few people can maintain assertive behaviour in all social contexts. Owen Hargie *et al.* (1987) draw attention to the need for knowledge. Assertive behaviour is unlikely to work effectively unless a person is clear about their rights and the social perceptions and meanings that are involved in any particular encounter. Assertion has to involve understanding the situation.

Although assertion is a skill, assertive behaviour will often depend on the following issues:

1 You have to understand the situation that you find yourself in. You have to be confident of your facts and your understanding of the other person's situation.

2 You have to be able to cope with your own inner feelings. Role can help with this – but whatever the situation you have to feel satisfied with yourself before you can be confident enough to be assertive.

3 You have to be able to act assertively – with the right non-verbal signals. Again, practice is very important here (don't smile if you're trying to be firm!)

4 You have to be able to act assertively with the right words and statements. Thinking this through in advance will help – you will need practice to become effective.

Using assertion effectively in a caring context will require a good knowledge of clients' rights, clients' needs and role boundaries. It will be important to avoid appearing aggressive; perhaps this will often be more important than appearing to be weak.

Using the right non-verbal signals and the right words and statements will depend on practice and experience. Practice and experience involve finding out what works in various contexts. This type of learning might involve learning through reinforcement. The main way of learning to be assertive is not through trial and error though. Trial and error can be a dangerous way of trying to get interpersonal behaviour right. Imitation learning – copying other people's behaviour – is a more effective way of learning. Besides imitation, use of imagination may be important. As suggested in Chapter 1, imagination can enable people to plan how to behave. So, cognitive, social learning theory and behaviourist perspectives can offer some guidance in understanding assertion. The best way to develop skills may be to undertake a specific training course in assertion.

Finally, coping with one's own inner feelings may involve using self-concept or other cognitive techniques to create confidence.

Using self-concept and other cognitive techniques to control emotion

Self-control may depend on being able to predict how we will behave if we feel threatened. There is evidence that individual confidence may often be linked to a person's ability to understand and evaluate themselves (Glynis Breakwell, 1992). It may be that self-confidence depends on having positive levels of self-esteem. People who are progressing towards self-actualisation, or people who feel content with their concept of self, may cope with conflict or aggression more easily than people who are uncertain of their own identity.

The development of a positive self-concept and the quest for self-actualisation may be lifelong tasks. Even so, there are some simple ideas which can help an individual to cope with aggression and stress.

Imagination provides a powerful tool for developing self-confidence. If an individual can imagine themselves doing and saying the right things, it can promote a belief in the person's competence. One reason people read novels, see films and so on, is to enable them to develop their own sense of self through imagination.

Another use of imagination is to review all the positive things about self. Before trying to cope with a stressful situation, a person might review their past achievements, recollect successes and times when they have coped with stress. For many people the most important thing to focus thought on may be the key features of personal identity. If family or friends are important to our sense of self, we might increase our sense of self-esteem by thinking about these people. If identity centres on religion we may have a saying or phrase which we repeat to ourselves. The saying may remind us of a sense of self and self-confidence.

A third idea is to be able to evaluate and analyse the thoughts that we use. Awareness of our own thinking processes or 'metacognitive knowledge' (p. 75) may empower an individual to question and check what they are doing.

For instance, if an important document has gone missing and an initial search fails, we could 'interpret' the situation as 'disastrous' – this is a catastrophe, someone must be punished, etc. This response causes stress. An alternative appraisal of this situation would be: 'This lost document presents an important problem – what can I do about it without becoming anxious or helpless?'

A version of this idea is called **thought stopping**. In thought stopping, the individual has to learn to recognise when they are becoming anxious or afraid. They then have to recognise their own inner conversation. Perhaps the careworker is thinking: 'It would be terrible if this person was to attack me – I might be humiliated, I might not cope, I'm worried, maybe I won't cope.' At this point the careworker thinks 'stop', and changes their thoughts to positive ideas about their self-concept. 'Stop' becomes conditioned to positive emotional feelings in the same way that 'relax' did when learning muscle relaxation. The real trick is to be able to understand our own personal thoughts, identify when they are letting us down and then deliberately change them using the 'stop' technique.

This technique will require a sense of self which can be separate from our minute by minute thoughts. The technique can also be taught. Here, the individual speaks their thoughts out loud, whilst the instructor talks about frightening situations. The instructor shouts 'stop' when the individual is becoming anxious. The theory is that this practical use of conversation will help the anxious individual to recognise their thought processes and learn to control them.

Using calming and conversational skills

Coping with aggression requires the ability to stay calm and encourage others to stay calm. Having achieved this stage it may be important to encourage talking and to try and establish a sense of common ground, a sense of trust, and maybe a sense of liking each other. Only after this second stage has been achieved will it be possible to negotiate a satisfactory solution to the issues that have sparked aggression.

Creating a calm atmosphere

In order to create a calm atmosphere it will be necessary to stay calm ourselves. This skill may depend on using the concept of work role, learning relaxation skills and having confidence in our own self-concept and assertion skills. If we can maintain self-control then we can attempt to influence an aggressive situation by using a range of verbal and non-verbal skills.

Non-verbal signals to improve calmness

Own posture should not display tension.

Movements should be slow and careful – not sharp or jerky.

Fixed expressions and eye-contact should not be too prolonged, and should be varied.

Allowance for 'personal space' should be made – back away if appropriate.

Facial expression should be 'serious' but relaxed.

Body posture should be at an angle towards the aggressive person – a 'facing

---

straight', 'face to face' posture is often understood as threatening; it may also make you more vulnerable to attack.

Arms should be dropped and relaxed; a gentle, slightly outward gesture with hands facing downwards may sometimes be used to signal calm by moving the hands gently up and down.

Mouth should be closed but relaxed.

Voice should be quiet but 'deliberate' and firm.

Verbal messages

It is vital to acknowledge the complaint or accusation that is being made; it makes it difficult for the other person to escalate the situation if their position is being listened to and understood. Although the other person may be deliberately trying to provoke you, it is important to prove that you are taking them seriously by reflecting back their messages. Perhaps the person says: 'You're always late, you don't care about me – you're too busy talking with the others.' Reflecting this back would involve saying something like: 'I'm sorry that you feel I don't care, but you are right that I do get very busy.'

The most important issue might be to try and keep the other person talking. Asking questions may help to achieve this. A carer's conversation should use supportive skills. The carer should be warm and sincere whilst trying to build an understanding of the situation. Praise and thanks for clarifying points may be useful in reducing any frustration that the other person may feel. Many people become aggressive because they don't know of any other way to cope. Reassurance that you have understood the problem may prevent aggression.

Before any serious issues can be discussed it will be very important to build a sense of safety and calm. Perhaps it will be possible to persuade the other person to agree to both of you sitting down to talk. Getting any kind of agreement is a very useful starting point for moving to the second stage of coping: trying to establish a sense of trust.

Creating trust

This stage involves trying to establish just a faint sense of common ground or liking each other. Instead of confronting the person, you are accepting the importance of their feelings, showing them that you really are trying to understand and yet being honest (and staying in control) by not agreeing to everything they say. As in the calming stage the key task is to prove that you are listening. It is also important to respect the other person's need for self-esteem. This can be done by meeting the person's need to feel important (although not their demands). Careful use of information about your own feelings, small pieces of information about your own history or difficulties can sometimes help to 'build bridges' and create a sense of similarity and safety. Although you may appear gentle, tolerant and supportive, it is vital that you do not agree with everything the other person demands. You have the very difficult task of offering support while using assertion skills to preserve your own control of the situation. The conversation needs to be kept going using questions, reinforcement and supportive listening.

Negotiating a solution - a problem-solving approach

This third stage might begin after it feels safe to raise the problems which have caused the aggression. This phase of 'sorting things out' might work in a similar way to dealing with conflicts that did not involve abuse and aggression. If conflicting viewpoints lead to argument, it may be possible to try and resolve the situation straight away. Where aggression is involved the stages of calming and building trust are likely to be necessary. These stages may be needed to create a suitably safe atmosphere for discussion and problem-solving work.

The possibilities for 'negotiation' or 'sorting things out' may be very different between different client groups. If the elder who is abusive also has dementia, then formal negotiation and problem solving may be inappropriate. Reminiscence work may be all that can be usefully done to resolve the aggression and leave everything OK when you walk away. Problem solving with a young child may be about creating a sense of fairness and coming to an agreement based on fair play.

The following ideas may be useful for working with arguments over beliefs and perceptions with adults and elders., They may also be useful when trying to resolve arguments with colleagues.

To begin with, it may be useful to try to clarify the issues involved. By carefully analysing issues it might be possible to offer a problem-solving approach – certain issues might have solutions and it is possible that the other person will feel that they are indeed having some of their needs met. Clarifying the issues may also enable you to present a range of alternatives to the other person. Alternatives often require some thought and it may be necessary to leave the person with your ideas for a short time.

Sometimes it is necessary to structure expectations; here you have decided what counts as a satisfactory outcome – perhaps your final answer has to be 'no'. Rather than confronting the person with this immediately, it may be better to slowly lead up to the expectation of 'no' by making the problem open, i.e. 'I understand your position and I'll try and see what I can do but it would be wrong to promise anything'; 'we can try but I'm not hopeful.'

Having listened and supported the other person, it may be possible to engage in formal negotiation, expecting the other person to behave in the same way. It may now be possible to forward your side of the argument and try and gain some (limited) sympathy for your point of view, i.e. 'I can see what you're saying, but can't you see my point of view? I'm not just arguing about rules, I have to defend other people's rights as well as yours.'

Carefully presented facts always help to support negotiation, and it may now be appropriate to introduce specific information to help the other person understand your view. If you take your time and present an objective, well-structured viewpoint which does not threaten the dignity of the other person, it may be possible to resolve the problem at this point. Usually, a degree of patience is required.

Following the presentation of your case it may be best to conclude by requesting delayed compliance, i.e. 'OK, well we don't have to agree now, I think we understand each other – why don't we talk tomorrow', or 'OK, you don't have to say yes or no now – think about it – think it through for a while.'

Negotiation requires an assertive attitude. Being assertive is different from 'winning'. A carer can always use their supportive skills to maintain the client's self-esteem needs. Successful negotiation is about coming to an agreed solution without anyone feeling that their dignity or self-concept has been undermined.

Using theory as a defence mechanism

Being able to understand a situation enables a carer to predict what might happen. If a carer can predict what the client might do, they may feel that their own personal skills are effective. If you can guess that the client will shout at you, you may be unhappy about being shouted at. On the other hand you may be pleased that you predicted things correctly. Your sense of self-esteem isn't threatened because you can be pleased with your ability to guess correctly!

Theory can support a worker's self-esteem by helping the careworker to understand events. Theory can be useful in helping us to balance beliefs and assumptions that exist in different situations. Sometimes people speak and behave as if all anger and all complaints are terrible things, to be avoided at all costs. The psychodynamic perspective would offer quite a different set of assumptions.

Freud believed that all creatures were motivated by a life drive, to grow, to develop and reproduce. As Freud developed his ideas, he came to believe that there was also an inbuilt self-destructive drive or death wish. When needs and desires go unmet or when they are suppressed, drive energy will build up in the individual. This energy might be directed outwardly as anger or aggression if it cannot be contained or released in a safer way. On the other hand, the energy might be directed inwardly in a self-destructive way. In self-destruction, the energy enables the individual to escape the horror of their situation through death. When viewed like this, aggression might seem a better alternative than depression or withdrawal.

Psychodynamic theory contains the idea that angry or aggressive outbursts will free the individual of emotional tension. The concept of catharsis is used to describe a discharge or release of emotional energy in a socially acceptable way. A person may be able to release their tension through taking part in aggressive or competitive sporting activity. They might be able to release the tension by watching a film that involves tension, horror or aggression. This release of tension is called a cathartic experience. The resident who became aggressive over the cup of tea might be achieving emotional release with their action. The problem is that this 'catharsis' is not acceptable to the careworker. The need to express anger, tension, frustration and fear might be acceptable to the careworker though! The issue would be to recognise what was happening and try to provide the resident with an opportunity to 'let off steam' safely. Conversation might be seen as a situation where the frustration and anger could be released in a socially acceptable way.

The idea that people need to release their energy and express their anger makes sense, but like all theory it will have a boundary. It will explain some things but not everything. Social learning theory would predict that there is a danger that people will learn to imitate behaviours which gain rewards. So, whilst an older resident might gain emotional release from watching a violent film, a child might simply learn to imitate the violence displayed on the film. Glynn Owens (1986) quotes evidence that opportunities for violent sport correlate with (or increase with) the levels of violence in a culture. Opportunities for releasing tension may also be opportunities to learn to be aggressive. Seeing aggression as a natural release of tension may help a careworker to cope. Seeing aggression as an acceptable form of behaviour because it may be 'natural' is very unwise. A careworker will need to be careful not to reinforce aggressive behaviour. Behavioural analysis (p. 43) may assist the careworker to ensure that they understand the results of their own behaviour.

All the theoretical perspectives provide ways of interpreting aggression and conflict.
- The neurobiological perspective draws attention to individual traits, to the physical state of a person, to illnesses and disabilities.
- The behaviourist perspective offers the concept of reinforcement as a way of understanding learning.

- Social learning theory expands this perspective and describes wider issues of learning through imitation in a social context.
- The cognitive perspective focuses attention on systems of meaning and assumptions that people operate from.
- The humanistic perspective offers ideas of self-concept and conversational techniques which might assist care work.

Making sense of any particular event might mean choosing concepts from a variety of perspectives. These concepts may help build an explanation. Skill in using concepts should result in personal self-confidence.

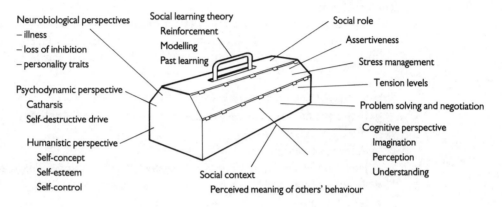

A tool kit of concepts to help make sense of aggression

Coping with stress

Abuse or aggression will automatically trigger a stress response in most people. The stress response is a biological reaction to enable an individual to cope with physical threat. The body is prepared to fight or run away. Heart rate increases, breathing becomes more rapid, digestion stops, muscles tense.

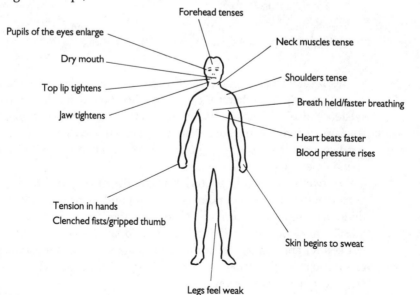

Recognise your own tension

Signs of feeling stressed

Usually the stress response may last for only ten or twenty minutes after an incident is over. Breathing and heart rate return to normal, digestion starts and muscles relax. The problems begin when the threat doesn't go away. Sometimes we may be concerned that we will have to face a difficult person again. Sometimes we may be afraid that an incident wasn't handled in the right way.

Some carers feel guilt at being abused! It is possible for a person to believe that as a carer they will always deserve respect. When aggression is experienced, the person assumes that they have caused it or that they have failed. Attitudes like this can lead to feelings of guilt.

Guilt, fear or anger can all keep a person stressed. In time, stress can damage the health of a careworker or lead to burn-out. According to Cherniss (1980), burn-out involves feelings of exhaustion and tension, and a change in attitude towards work.

Indicators of burn-out adapted from Cherniss:
- High resistance to work every day (not wanting to go there – not wanting to be there or do the work).
- A sense of failure.
- Feelings of anger, resentment, and negativity to clients and colleagues.
- Feelings of guilt and blame towards self and others.
- Isolation and withdrawal.
- Feeling tired and exhausted all day.
- Stereotyping clients and other people.
- Inability to really listen to other people.
- Suspicion and fear of other people.
- Poor sleep patterns.
- Frequent colds and illnesses leading to time off.
- Frequent headaches and stomach upsets.
- Alcohol abuse.
- Conflict with others.
- Rigid thinking.

Glynis Breakwell (1989) notes that carers 'have a tendency to avoid using the services of other carers' (p. 75) when seeking help following an attack. She continues to identify the existence of a tendency to 'blame the victim' amongst some social workers, nurses and teachers. It may be the case that tired and stressed colleagues find it easier to ignore conflict and aggression, and to blame those who end up on the receiving end rather than spend time in supporting victims.

Breakwell also points out that 'blaming the careworker' for being a victim also maintains the idea that careworkers can control and manage all situations. It is important to think in terms of the enormous complexity of human behaviour; to think about the almost infinite range of explanations for an individual's behaviour. Of course, careworkers cannot control and manage every possible situation. It is not appropriate to assume that a careworker should always be able to understand, cope with, or control every source of anger, conflict or aggression.

Stress may become a problem for carers because of the distress of clients, stressed colleagues at work, burn-out, and the assumption that carers should always be able to cope. There is a range of stress management techniques that individuals can try. Learning to use individual stress control skills is only part of the picture though.

Alan Mclean (1979) points out that coping with stress involves at least three major issues. Firstly, there is the nature and intensity of the stress – being physically attacked is usually more stressful than receiving a complaint. Secondly, there is the social and environmental context of the individual. Do you have support from colleagues, support in other social relationships, resources, money, time, clear work roles, and so on? Thirdly, how vulnerable to stress is the individual? What strength of self-concept or identity does the individual have, what state of health, what personality factors, what concepts and thought systems? What stress management skills and stability zones does the individual have?

The three areas come together to enable a prediction of coping or failing to cope with long-term stress.

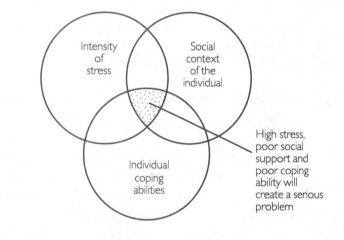

Factors which may influence how stressed an individual becomes

The size of the circle indicates the intensity of the problem. A large overlap indicates a risk of not coping. A small overlap or a lack of overlapping problems might suggest that stress can be coped with.

Reflective activity

A quick stress check for work or placement settings
Give yourself a mark out of five for each question, with One meaning that everything is almost as good as it could be, and Five meaning that things are almost as bad as you can imagine. Three means neither good or bad, or no real opinion. Add your scores at the end of each question area.

Area 1 Stress at work/on placement
1 How clear are you about what is expected of you at work?
2 Are you ever bored with your work?
3 Do you feel that there is far too much to do in the time you have?
4 Do you come into conflict with colleagues or clients?

5 Do you feel in control of/or on top of your work, do you enjoy work?

6 How confident do you feel at work?

Area 2 Support at work/on placement

1 How friendly are the colleagues that you work with?

2 How much advice and guidance or supervision do you get at work?

3 Do you have friends or family you can discuss work issues with?

4 Do you usually know where to go and who to ask when there is a problem at work?

5 Do you feel that the work you do is worthwhile and useful?

6 Do your colleagues expect you to have useful ideas and do they listen to your ideas?

Area 3 Personal coping strategies

1 If you feel stressed, is there somewhere or some activity you can always go to, in order to lose the stress?

2 Do you feel you can cope assertively with difficult work situations?

3 When you think about your past life, how confident do you feel about your abilities?

4 When you think about your life, how happy are you with being the person that you see yourself as?

5 Do you feel that you worry a lot about work – can you control these worries or do they keep coming into your mind?

6 How far can you control your own emotions of fear, tension and anger?

- Which area did you score highest on? What can you do in the long term to reduce stress, to increase support, or to improve your own coping abilities?

- Discuss the outcome of this stress survey with a tutor or supervisor. How could you develop this into a study of coping with caring in a specific care context?

Stress, support and supervision at work are key themes for the next chapters. In terms of coping with stress at work, support and supervision will often be more important than personal coping strategies. A few ideas on personal coping are listed here for reference. Many of the ideas are difficult to build into a lifestyle just from reading a book. Usually, a person has to have a friendship network or join an activity group in order to really learn these skills. Even exercise can sometimes be difficult to keep up if you try and do it entirely alone without any social reinforcement.

Stress management techniques

Stability zones

A first idea for stress management is to develop stability zones. The idea of having a stability zone is to have a safe place where we can control our tension levels and take time out from stress. The need for personal 'zones' of stability was suggested by Tanya Arroba and Kim James (1987). They suggest six main kinds of 'zone' which might help an individual to relax and feel safe.

Places
A physical location where you can expect to be free of stress and learn to control personal tension.

Values and beliefs

Thought systems which reinforce self-image and self-esteem. Reflection on values about identity and life can enable an individual to relabel or reinterpret life experience. Time taken to reflect on values can enable an individual to gain psychological control of the stress response.

Things

Possessions and objects become 'associated' (or 'conditioned') with feelings and thoughts. Objects can become a talisman, where simply looking at/or touching the object causes a feeling of relaxation.

People

Personal relationships provide a source of identity and self-esteem for many people. As for 'values and beliefs', friendship and relationships provide a context for a 'sense of self' which can enable people to gain psychological control of physiological reactions.

Organisations

As for 'people' above, an organisation can provide a sense of 'belonging' or personal recognition. Recognition develops self-worth, which in turn helps gain control of the psychological triggers of stress.

Activities

Developing skills, experiencing challenges, learning, and exercising can provide instances of diversions and alternative stresses. 'Alternative stress' may help an individual to lose the effects of involuntary stress.

Arroba and James (1987) argue that each individual requires a range of the above 'stability zone' activities. Concentrating stress management skills in one area results in vulnerability. If self-esteem and coping are concentrated perhaps in family life, then loss of family role results in stress. In addition to this stress, the loss of family removes the individual's resources for successful adjustment to stress.

Other personal stress management techniques

Progressive muscle relaxation

This is a training regime originated by a Dr Jacobson as long ago as 1929. The technique requires many sessions of alternatively contracting and relaxing specific sets of body muscles. In time, an individual can control their muscles and can bring on muscle relaxation at will. Nowadays, trainees often learn to associate a specific word like 'relax' with a state of self-induced relaxation. The ability to consciously control muscle tension should inhibit (or stop) the stress response. A person who is good at muscle relaxation might make a conscious decision not to experience stress.

Problems: Some authors argue that the technique can be self-taught, but some people might not recognise their own muscle states. There can be problems with getting enough practice to learn the technique. Yoga would provide a similar set of skills and it may be easier to join a group and be taught yoga.

Biofeedback

Electrical gadgets can be used to measure 'galvanic skin response' or even muscle tension. Where a measure of tension can be obtained, it provides a baseline for learning to control tension. Basically, most biofeedback involves monitoring personal stress levels, while the individual seeks to reduce these levels with personal attempts at relaxation. By reducing tension at will, a person can gain a feeling of control over stress.

Problems: The novelty of a monitor puts some people off and upsets attempts to relax. For others there is the possibility of becoming stuck, or bored with the gadget – a bit like exercise bikes! Irregular practice may offer only minimal gains.

Meditation

Meditation will induce a deep state of relaxation via concentration of attention on a simple focus. The focus might be the sound of a word, an object, a light source (candle), or one's own breathing or heart rate. There are various versions of the process, but all versions involve a passive attitude and what might be described as a mild trance of concentration. This concentration is perhaps similar to concentrating on music at a concert: you drift with the experience, concentrating but not thinking in any analytic way. Meditation need not be associated with any religious or mystic belief systems.

Problems: Some people have difficulty with getting started; meditation can be difficult to learn alone despite its individual nature. Like all skills the approach takes time. It also requires uninterrupted use of a quiet space on a regular basis – this has to be available.

Emergency relaxation

A technique suggested by Jane Madders (1981) which concentrates on breathing techniques, taking one component from the progressive muscle relaxation approach – that of relaxing the muscles associated with breathing. When feeling stressed:

1 Say or think 'Stop!'
2 Breathe in deeply and breathe out slowly. Whilst breathing out, relax hands and shoulders by dropping the shoulders and allowing the hands to hang limp.
3 Breathe in deeply again, and relax jaw and mouth when breathing out.
4 Take two small quiet breaths and continue the task in hand at a calmer and more controlled pace. Continue to check for tension – like other relaxation skills, this technique requires practice in non-stressful situations before it will be useful.

Use of imagination/ideation

A form of self-hypnosis where scenes are imagined. Pre-recorded tapes can be used to induce a trance-like tranquillity. Some people can achieve similar effects with music.

Problems: Some people find it easier to relax this way than others. The technique may require time and practice, if it is to become a useful 'stability zone'.

Physical exercise

Physical exercise doesn't stop the stress response directly but it may enable a stressed person to turn the stress response off! Vigorous exercise provides an outlet for the results of stress. Besides improving general health, exercise may burn up the fats and sugars released into the bloodstream, as well as remove other harmful side-effects of the stress response.

Problems: Risks of over-exercising when unfit, problems with time, and the risk of becoming addicted to exercise.

Desensitisation

When individuals need help with fear, rather than stress as such, it may be possible to seek help from a professionally qualified psychologist. Desensitisation is one form of help which is aimed at enabling an individual to unlearn a fear reaction.

Desensitisation usually starts with an analysis of a feared situation – perhaps, for example, a fear (or phobia) of using a lift. Things associated with lifts (e.g. walking past a lift) are analysed. The person with the fear is then taught relaxation techniques.

Desensitisation might begin with imagining minor fears and learning to relax while imagining them. Soon the person can imagine their worst fear and stay calm and relaxed. Following this stage, the person would continue with desensitisation in real life. Relaxation would be associated with each aspect of the feared situation (using the lift). Eventually the person should learn to relax, rather than panic when using the lift. Desensitisation is now complete.

Desensitisation could be tried in relation to any feared situation including coping with aggression. Expert clinical help might be needed in order to use this technique safely and effectively.

Affectionless psychopathy

Bowlby theorised that maternal deprivation – during a critical period – could create 'psychopathy' in adolescents. Affectionless psychopathy involves a lack of care for others and an inability to express affection for others.

Aggression

Behaviour which promotes the interests of an individual or group while denying or damaging the interests of others. Aggressive attitudes involve concentrating on personal needs and wants, and ignoring or opposing the needs and wants of others.

Assertiveness

The ability to clearly and openly explain personal needs and wants while considering and understanding the needs and wants of others. Assertive attitudes involve listening to, and negotiating with other people.

Attachment

Bowlby theorised that special bonds between mother and baby might develop in early infancy. Failure to develop these bonds might seriously disrupt the child's development. Research evidence suggests that babies can form multiple attachments; not just with the 'mother'.

Attitudes

A tendency to react to issues in a set way. Attitudes are based on the beliefs and belief systems that an individual has developed. Attitudes will influence individual emotional feelings and how a person understands new information or experiences.

Attribution

To attribute, or draw conclusions about, the causes of other people's behaviour.

Behaviourism

A psychological perspective that tries to understand human (and animal) actions in relation to past learning. In 'radical' behaviourism the environment is assumed to control behaviour through conditioned learning processes. Social behaviourism takes a broader view of learning, emphasising cognitive ability. Behaviourism provides the foundation for the social learning perspective.

Behaviour modification

A training process which relies on the use of reinforcement (or operant conditioning). New 'desirable' behaviours are reinforced sometimes with the intention of replacing other patterns of behaviour. The approach is based on the behaviourist perspective.

Catharsis

A term used in the psychodynamic perspective to describe a release of emotional energy or 'letting off steam'. A cathartic experience involves a release of inner tension during some activity or event in a way that the individual regards as socially acceptable.

Chaos theory

A new approach to science and scientific study which sees events as evolving out of chaos. Chaos theory denies that everything has a 'cause'. People interpret events as having causes, but these may be no more than patterns which have emerged from underpinning chaos.

Cognitive development

The development of thinking systems. Cognitive development in children was studied by Piaget (1896–1980). He believed that thought developed as a consequence of biological motivation and learning. His theories are often explained using a 'four-stage' model. This model of child development is not always accepted as a completely satisfactory theory however.

Cognitive perspective

A psychological approach which focuses on the processes involved in perception, thinking and the development of knowledge systems. Human behaviour is often explored with reference to processes such as memory, problem solving, language and concept formation. The perspective can often be combined with other perspectives to provide deeper explanations of behaviour.

Concepts

Concepts are mental categories which enable people to make sense of the world. Concepts enable us to simplify the world and use language to classify it. Concepts also enable prediction of future events. Concepts can be combined to produce theories.

Concrete-operational period

The third stage in Piaget's analysis of cognitive development – perhaps about seven to twelve years of age. The main features are the ability to de-centre and to use 'concrete' logical operations.

Conditioning

A type of learning experience described within the behaviourist perspective. Classical (or Pavlovian) conditioning involves learning to associate experiences together, i.e. to learn to associate a bell with the arrival of food. Operant (or Skinnerian) conditioning involves learning to repeat behaviours which are reinforced (have a pleasurable outcome).

Consistency

The degree to which people tend to be consistent in their behaviour across different social contexts and situations. In general, research indicates that social context plays a major role in influencing behaviour. People adapt to their situation or context.

Critical period

A particular period of early infancy in animals and humans when relationships or 'bonds' are formed between the infant and the mother, according to Bowlby's theory.

Desensitisation

A learning process aimed at unlearning a fear, or unlearning a fear reaction to some situation. Desensitisation usually involves association or conditioned learning, where a relaxation response becomes associated with a previously feared situation.

Discrimination

The original meaning of the word is to be able to distinguish between things or situations. In a care context, discrimination usually implies that some people are denied the same quality of care or opportunities as certain other people because they belong to some predefined group or class. Discrimination would occur where members of certain races or one gender receive better treatment than others.

Ego

A term used in the psychodynamic perspective to describe 'the reality principle'. The ego is responsible for channelling drive energy into behaviour. The ego may correspond with the term 'identity' in other perspectives to some extent.

Electra complex

A female version of the Oedipus complex within psychodynamic theory. The girl forms an attachment to the father which has to be subsequently abandoned. The father's values become internalised as a result of the resolution of the 'complex'.

Emotion

A general term which covers mental, perceptual and physiological reactions to events. Different perspectives make different assumptions about the significance of learning, physiology and cognitive processes when attempting to explain emotional reactions.

Empowerment

To enable others to control their own lives, make their own decisions and achieve positive self-esteem and identities. Care workers might focus care values on the concept of client empowerment.

Extroversion

The opposite of introversion. A dimension of temperament, according to Hans Eysenck. In Eysenck's theory, extroverts are stimulus hungry and seek novel and exciting experiences.

Formal operations

The final stage of cognitive development in Piaget's theory. Piaget believed that after the age of eleven or twelve, children would begin to use deductive logic and abstract reasoning. It is widely accepted that there is great variation in logical and abstract reasoning ability and that many people do not develop these skills.

Genetics–environment debate

A historical debate in psychology about the relative power of genetics and learning to influence human personality and intelligence. Both factors are generally accepted to exert an influence. The balance of influence only becomes a key debate where causal explanations are looked for (see chaos theory).

Helplessness

A learned condition where an individual gives up and withdraws from attempts to control their life or circumstances. Helplessness may be a consequence of disempowerment; and of care where the staff control their clients with institutional approaches.

Humanistic perspective

A perspective that explores human behaviour in terms of personal needs. The ultimate need is for self-actualisation or fulfilment of human potential. The perspective is particularly associated with the work of Carl Rogers and Abraham Maslow.

Id

A term used in psychodynamic theory to describe the 'powerhouse' of drive energy which motivates behaviour. The id is the pleasure principle – instinctive drives which demand to be satisfied.

Ideal self

A view of self as you would like to be. A concept of self as you think you ought to be. The term is used within the humanistic perspective.

Identity

An understanding of self. Personal identity might include hidden and inner understandings of self. Social identity might include group memberships which influence others' understanding of you.

Introversion

The opposite of extroversion. Hans Eysenck used the term to identify a feature of temperament where an individual is easily over-stimulated. Introverts are theorised to be people who will try to avoid large amounts of excitement.

Maternal deprivation

Bowlby's theory suggested a critical period of mother/child contact which was required during the first five years of life. A continuous break in mother/child contact of more than one week might result in 'maternal deprivation' and emotional problems in later life.

Metacognition

The ability to understand your own thinking processes. Metacognition is more than simply being able to 'reflect' on ideas. Metacognitive knowledge involves thinking about the way you use reflective skills. Metacognition might be a more important focus than 'formal operations' when trying to understand cognitive development.

Monotropy

Bowlby's belief that young children need constant care by one main naturally qualified carer – the mother. If maternal care was not provided, Bowlby predicted lasting psychological damage would happen to the child.

Motivation

The term comes from a Latin word which means to move. Motivation is a broad term meaning what moves behaviour or what creates or causes behaviour. The perspectives covered in Chapter 2 all make different assumptions about what motivates people to act.

Neurobiological perspective

A perspective which tries to find explanations for behaviour by exploring the workings of our physiological systems.

NVQ value base

A professional basis for delivering empowering care. It includes anti-discriminatory practice, the maintenance of confidentiality, maintenance of clients' rights and choice, respect for clients' identity and beliefs; and the ability to value clients with appropriate conversation.

Oedipus complex

A term used in Freudian (psychodynamic) theory. The male equivalent to the Electra complex. The boy develops an attachment to the mother which then has to be abandoned, causing the boy to adopt his mother's value system.

Perception

The process of making sense of information from our senses (sight, hearing, touch, etc.). Perception involves past learning, expectations and assumptions as well as the ability to 'sense things'.

Personality

A broad term which covers the psychological qualities of an individual which appear to provide a stable influence on the individual's behaviour. Personality would include concepts such as self-concept, traits, temperament and cognition.

Perspectives

Ways of trying to make sense of behaviour. Perspectives are much more fundamental than theories. Perspectives cannot be disproved! Perspectives make assumptions about the nature of the questions to be asked about human behaviour.

Prejudice

Literally pre-judgement. Prejudice relates to fixed attitudes which may result in discrimination and disempowerment for members of specific groups or classes.

Pre-operational

The second stage in Piaget's interpretation of cognitive development (approximately two to seven years of age). The child learns to use language and symbolic thought. 'Egocentrism' and 'centration' feature at this stage.

Primacy and recency effect

'Primacy' is used in interpersonal perception to identify the idea that the first thing we find out about someone will make the greatest impression. Recency is the idea that we often remember the last thing about a situation most clearly. Primacy and recency suggest that impressions of others will be most strongly influenced by the first and last information we have about them.

Privation

Michael Rutter's term for a lack of some support or relationship for a child. Privation might relate to the non-existence of emotional bonding rather than the interruption in a relationship which would be 'deprivation'.

Problem-solving

When used in the context of resolving conflict and aggression this term relates to the negotiation or persuasion phase of coping. The approach is possible where individuals assume an assertive attitude, rather than an aggressive or submissive (weak) attitude.

Psychodynamic perspective

A view of human behaviour based on assumptions about internal drives and components of mind. Sigmund Freud originated the perspective although many subsequent authors have developed the approach. Psychoanalysis – Freud's talking cure – based on an emphasis on the unconscious, is a key therapeutic tool used within the perspective.

Reinforcement

Sometimes called operant conditioning. Reinforcement strengthens certain behaviours that lead to desirable outcomes. Reinforcement is a central part of behaviourist learning theory.

Relaxation

A stress reduction technique that involves learning to control personal physiology.

Role

Patterns of behaviour which are performed in order to fit other people's social expectations.

Self-actualisation

A term used within the humanistic perspective to describe the ultimate need for personal fulfilment. Self-actualisation involves the idea that 'what you can be – you must be'. Self-actualisation involves becoming what you have the potential to become.

Self-concept

An individual's concept or understanding of themself. The self-concept is likely to include private or hidden ideas about self as well as aspects of social identity.

Self-control or staying calm

A learned skill for coping in situations involving aggression or high levels of emotional reaction. The skill may involve the use of imagination, self-concept, theories and relaxation techniques.

Self-esteem

The degree of value that a person puts on their understanding of themself. How a person values themselves. High self-esteem may help a person to feel confident. Low self-esteem may lead to depression and unhappiness.

Self-image

The perceived view of self that a person develops within their social context.

Sensori-motor

Piaget's first stage of cognitive development (birth to two years). In the sensori-motor stage, infants learn to associate perception with their own activity. Children learn to understand the permanence of objects during this stage.

Separation anxiety

Separation anxiety relates to Bowlby's theory that young children separated from their mother will suffer a 'grief' type of reaction.

Social context

The setting for group and social influences on individual learning. There is a growing body of knowledge that suggests that social context may have a central influence on the understanding of human behaviour. Social context may be considered as another perspective for understanding behaviour.

Social learning perspective

An approach to understanding human behaviour which builds on the foundations of behaviourism, but rejects the radical behaviourist view that people are simply controlled by 'operants'. Social learning theory accepts the role of cognition and imagination in influencing learning.

Stability zones

A term used in stress management theory by Arroba and James. Stability zones are places, people or things that create a sense of safety and relaxation.

Stereotyping

Classifying objects or people together using limited or fixed criteria and then failing to perceive individual differences. Stereotyping is like typecasting or labelling.

Super ego

A term used in psychodynamic theory to describe the 'morality principle'. The super ego, along with the ego and id, form the main components of mind within the psychodynamic perspective.

Temperament

The way in which biological influences create behavioural styles within an individual. Introversion and extroversion are theorised as being a dimension of temperament according to Hans Eysenck.

Trait

A stable quality within a person that is theorised to influence behaviour. Traits are theorised to cause tendencies to respond in particular ways. Introversion and extroversion could be described as traits, as could a tendency to perform well in group situations.

Values

Learned principles or thought systems which guide individual choice and decision-making processes.

SECTION ONE – References and further reading

References

Argyle, M., *The Psychology of Interpersonal Behaviour* 2nd edn (Penguin, 1990)

Arroba, T. and James, K., *Pressure at Work* (McGraw-Hill, 1987)

Bandura, A., *Social Learning Theory* (Prentice Hall, 1977)

Bandura, A., *Social Foundations of Thought and Action: a Social Cognitive Theory* (Englewood Cliffs: Prentice Hall, 1986)

Bartlett, F.C., *Remembering* (Cambridge University Press, 1932)

Bowlby, J., *Attachment and Loss*, Vol. 1 *Attachment* (Tavistock, 1969)

Brayne, C. and Ames, D., 'The Epidemiology of Mental Disorders in Old Age' in Gearing *et al.* (ed.), *Mental Health Problems in Old Age* (Wiley, 1988)

Breakwell, G., *Facing Physical Violence* (BPS and Routledge, 1989)

Brown, H., *People, Groups and Society* (OUP, 1985)

Cattell, R., *The Scientific Analysis of Personality* (Penguin, 1965)

Cherniss, C., *Staff Burnout* (Sage Publications, 1980)

Cohen, D., *Piaget – Critique and Reassessment* (Croom Helm, 1983)

Cook, M., *Levels of Personality* (Holt, Rinehart and Winston, 1984)

Cooley, C.H., *Human Nature and Social Order* (Scribners, 1902)

Deaux, K., 'Personalising Identity and Socialising Self' in G. Breakwell (ed.), *Social Psychology of Identity and the Self Concept* (Surrey University Press, 1992)

Donaldson, M., *Children's Minds* (Fontana, 1978)

Eysenck, H., *Fact and Fiction in Psychology* (Pelican, 1965)

Flavell, J.H., 'Metacognition and Cognitive Monitoring' (1979) *American Psychologist* 34, 906–11

Fox, N., 'Attachment of Kibbutz Infants to Mother and Metapelet' (1977) *Journal of Child Development* 48, 1, 228–39

Freud, S. (1900), *The Interpretation of Dreams*, Standard edn (Chatto and Windus)

Freud, S. (1905), *Three Essays on the Theory of Sexuality* Standard edn (Chatto and Windus)

Gagne, R. (1977), *The Conditions of Learning* 3rd edn (Holt Saunders)

Gleick, J., *Chaos Making a New Science* (Cardinal, 1987)

Goffman, E., *The Presentation of Self in Everyday Life* (Pelican, 1971 (first version published 1959))

Hargie, O., Saunders, C., Dickson, D., *Source Skills in Interpersonal Communication* 2nd edn (Croom Helm and Brookline Books, 1987)

Hartshorne, H. and May, M., *Studies in the Nature of Character* (Macmillan, 1930)

Herbert, M., *Behavioural Treatment of Problem Children* (Academic Press, 1981)

Hughes, M., *Egocentrism in Pre-school Children* (Edinburgh University, 1975)

Jacques, A., *Understanding Dementia* (Churchill Livingstone, 1988)

Kelley, H.H., 'The Warm Cold Variable in First Impressions of People' (1950) *Journal of Personality* 18, 431–9

Lloyd, P. *et al.*, *Introduction to Psychology* (Fontana, 1984)

Luchins, A., 'Primacy–Recency in Impression Formation' in C. Howland (ed.), *The Order of Presentation in Persuasion* (Yale University Press, 1957)

Luft, J., *Group Processes: An Introduction to Group Dynamics* (Mayfield, 1970)

Madders, J., *Stress and Relaxation* 3rd edn (Optima, 1981)

Mclean, A., *Work-Stress* (Addison-Wesley, 1979)

Mead, G.H., *Mind, Self and Society* (University of Chicago Press, 1934)

Minard, R.D., 'Race Relations in the Pocohontas Coalfield' (1952) *Journal of Social Issues* 8, 29–44

Mischel, W., *Personality and Assessment* (Wiley, 1968)

Owens, R.G., 'Handling Strong Emotions' in O. Hargie (ed.), *A Handbook of Communication Skills* (Croom Helm, 1986)

Rakos, R., 'Asserting and Confronting' in O. Hargie (ed.), *A Handbook of Communication Skills* (Croom Helm, 1986)

Roth, I. in I. Roth and J. Frisby, *Perception and Representation* (OUP, 1986)

Rutter, M., *Maternal Deprivation Reassessed* 2nd edn (Penguin, 1981)

Ryle, G., *The Concept of Mind* (Penguin, 1973 (first published 1949))

Sapir, E., 'The Status of Linguistics as a Science' (1929) *Language* 5, 207–14

Seligman, M., *Helplessness* (W.H. Freeman & Co., 1975)

Sherif, M. and Sherif, C.W., *Groups in Harmony and Tension* (1953)

Sherif, M. *et al.*, *Experimental Study of Positive and Negative Intergroup Attitudes Between Experimentally Produced Groups* (Norman, University of Oklahoma, 1955)

Sherif, M. *et al.*, *Intergroup Co-operation and Competition* (Norman, University of Oklahoma, 1961)

Smith, E., 'Concepts and Thought' in E. Sterberg and E. Smith (eds), *The Psychology of Human Thought* (Cambridge University Press, 1988)

Tajfel, H. *et al.*, 'Social Categorisation and Intergroup Behaviour' (1971) *European Journal of Social Psychology* Vol. 2, 149–78

Tizard, B. and Hodges, J., 'The Effect of Early Institutional Rearing on the Development of Eight Year Old Children' (1978) *Journal of Child Psychology and Psychiatry* 12, 99–118

Tomlin, S., *Abuse of Elderly People* (Report from the British Geriatrics Society, 1989)

Wharf, B.L., 'The Relation of Habitual Thought and Behaviour to Language' in Spier (ed.), *Language, Culture and Personality* (University of Utah Press, 1941)

Recommended further reading

Atkinson, R.L., Atkinson, R.C., Smith, E.E., Bem, D.J., *Introduction to Psychology* 10th edn (Harcourt, Brace, Jovanovich, 1990)

Birch, A. and Malim, T., *Developmental Psychology* (Intertext Ltd., 1988)

Breakwell, G., *Facing Physical Violence* (BPS and Routledge, 1989)

Hays, N., *Foundations of Psychology* (Routledge, 1994)

For reference

Gross, R.D. *Psychology* 2nd edn (Hodder and Stoughton, 1992)

5 Working with people in care organisations

What is covered in this chapter

- Caring
- Groups
- Teams
- Leadership
- Work role
- Characteristics of a good group member

This chapter aims to provide deeper understanding of the factors which enable people to work together effectively in a group. You will be encouraged to critically review a number of group situations to enable you to collect evidence required by BTEC Unit 13.

Emphasis on the uniqueness of individuals has been a key feature of earlier chapters. This chapter will enable you to develop this way of thinking, and to gain an understanding of the different roles and processes involved in working in care organisations.

Caring

Reflective activity

Imagine that you are discussing your future career with a well-meaning friend. 'So you want to be a carer?' your friend says with some misgivings. 'Yes' you reply with conviction, but what is a carer and what makes you feel confident that this is the right career move for you?

Socialisation

In many cultures, caring is seen by some as a natural extension of a woman's role. Those who hold such views see a woman's role purely as a home maker and the person with responsibility for caring for others. Sociologists define culture as being the ways in which a baby learns the acceptable way to behave in the society he or she is born into. Watching and listening to those around them in its early life, a baby quickly adopts the behaviour patterns it observes, coming to accept the attitudes and values expressed by significant others in its early life as the way the world is.

Behaviour which is seen by adults as acceptable is reinforced and deviant behaviour disapproved of. Reinforcement of socially acceptable behaviour may be by a smile, a cuddle or words of encouragement. Reinforcement of behaviour seen as anti-social may be by words of disapproval; often a severe tone is adopted accompanied by a stern face.

You may have noted in an earlier chapter that reinforcement does have its pitfalls! You may wish to re-read the section on behaviourism and consider the approach you would take to assist a young child to learn, for example, socially acceptable eating habits in your own culture. Do make sure that you are reinforcing the behaviour you want the child to adopt though!

Gender roles are also learnt in early life and are therefore a product of socialisation, as pointed out by sociologist Ann Oakley (1972) who built on the work of psychoanalyst Dr Robert Stoller (1968).

To gain a deeper understanding, you may wish to review the chapter on gender in any good sociology textbook, for example *Sociology Themes and Perspectives* by M. Haralambos (3rd edition, 1991), Chapter 9, p. 521.

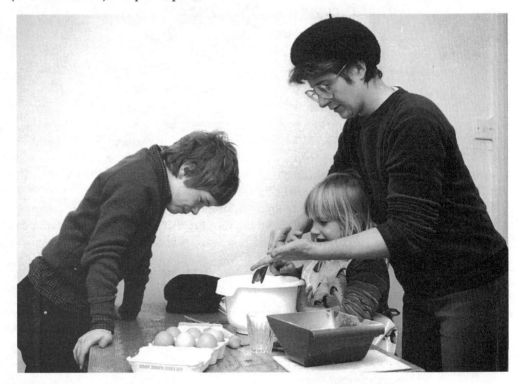

Many cultures see caring as a natural extension of a woman's role

In those cultures where the gender role of women is seen as that of a home maker and child rearer above all else, it is possible to see that that same culture might expect the role of a carer to be merely an extension of a woman's role, i.e. to provide assistance to others in need of support in some way. Perhaps this is an explanation for the majority of carers in the past in Britain being women and to some extent this remains true today.

Reflective activity

What do you think about this issue? Do these statistics demonstrate current social views regarding gender roles? You may wish to discuss this with a friend or perhaps with staff in a care setting to gain their perceptions.

Whether you are a male or female carer (and it is important to have both, since both men and women need professional help from carers!), the knowledge and skills that you require are complex and should not be underestimated. Common sense may well play a part, but to be effective as a carer you require an understanding of yourself and others.

Motivation

It may be argued that each of us enters work for a variety of reasons: from the very practical motivation to earn money to live on, to a far deeper motivation factor to meet a personal need. You may wish to refer to Hull (1943), Maslow (1943), Skinner (1953), Ausubel (1969), Cattell and Child (1975) to review the range of theories of motivation.

Maslow, for example, sees the need for 'esteem' as about confidence in self on the one hand and the wish for respect from others and therefore prestige on the other. Do you think that this is one of the factors which motivates people to work in the care field? Perhaps providing a service for others at a time of need helps carers to achieve the personal esteem needs as described by Maslow.

Consider also Ausubel's theory of motivation to achieve, in terms of care. This may provide a useful explanation of a carer's behaviour. First, the cognitive drive requires a carer to have knowledge of biology, social systems, basic psychology, sophisticated communication and interpersonal skills, to name but a few. Increasing one's understanding of the needs of others and learning ways to support them, surely give greater confidence to a carer as they become more knowledgeable and experienced.

In turn this will lead to the second part, 'self enhancement', i.e. increased knowledge about the role of the carer and increased understanding of others. This leads to greater confidence in one's ability to 'do a good job'.

The ability to do a good job brings approval from others: whether it is through a client having confidence in the carer or a senior giving increased responsibility to a member of staff. Ausubel called this 'affiliation'.

This may be expressed in a simple diagram:

Increased knowledge – Increased confidence – Increased satisfaction

Reflective activity

How does this apply to you? What is it about you as an individual that encourages you to consider a career in caring? Perhaps it is the reinforcement you have received from others when you have gone to help them; for example, 'I can always talk to you, you listen and seem to understand'; or 'I do not know where you get the patience to work with people like that!'; or 'You are so good with people!' Such comments make us feel good and we take them on board to incorporate them into the way that we see ourselves. In this way we are meeting a basic need to be accepted by others which helps to raise our self-esteem.

Take some time to think through the motives that encourage you to consider this career. You could make a list which might include any practical experiences of care you have been involved in and also comments made to you by others which have encouraged you. You may also find it helpful to look again at your attempt at Johari's window in Chapter 1, to help you to determine the factors which have motivated you to take this career step.

If you have briefly considered the issues of motivation, you may begin to gain a clearer understanding of yourself.

- List the qualities you have which you are able to use to work effectively with clients. List a minimum of eight and then place them in order of importance.
- You may wish to ask another person to look at your list. Ask them to decide what

the rank order should be if they were one of your clients. You may well find some surprising answers, which you should discuss with your partner. This will enable you to gain a better understanding of how they perceive your role to meet their needs.

It is important to remember that caring is a specialised career because every person you work alongside will be different. The difference will be biological and social. This will also mean that every individual will have a different perception of themselves and you as their carer. This will affect the way that they will expect you to behave and indeed the way that they will behave when with you.

Individual differences

Chapter 2 describes how difficult it is to identify the causes of behaviour. Yet it is important to appreciate individual differences and to try and gain an insight and understanding of life from the individual client's perspective. Understanding may lead you to empathise with an individual.

Reflective activity

Imagine that you have been asked to escort an elderly woman from her house to a residential home where she has decided to live because of failing health. You could decide that your role is rather like that of a delivery agent collecting a product from point A and safely delivering it to point B. Success may then be seen as the safe arrival at point B of the 'package' – your job is completed or is it?

Empathy

Caring is about being sensitive to others' needs, not just about achieving results as above. A sensitive carer will be aware of the possible emotional conflict facing this woman. She has had to make a big decision to give up her home and to move into a strange environment, however friendly and helpful the people there may seem. She may be relieved that she has felt able to take the decision to move, or she may be feeling helpless in finding that she has no other viable option. She may well feel that her role as independent home owner is over and be unsure of any new role in her new environment. Her perception about who she is and her value as an individual may be in question, i.e. her identity is threatened.

The way you interact with her as she closes her front door and travels to the centre with you will make a great deal of difference to her when she is perhaps feeling very vulnerable. You will need to reassure her that she is valued as an individual and demonstrate that by empowering her to take responsibility for herself. Respecting her culture as an individual is an important issue, as is every other aspect of her life, so ask her, and do not assume anything! Give the client time, instead of being brusque and rushing her; reassure her of her independence in her new home. Listen to her or perhaps just sit in silence allowing her time to make some emotional adjustments.

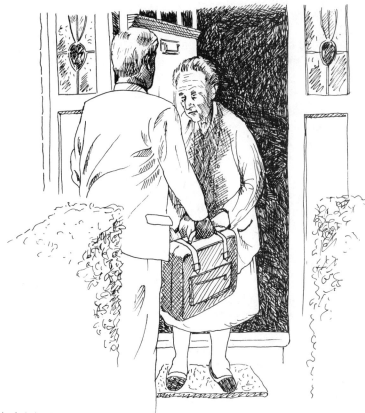

Caring and admission to care

It is not easy to decide what is going to be the best way to support a person especially if you do not really know them very well. Be aware of their possible thoughts and feelings and behave sensitively towards them. By watching the non-verbal communication as well as listening and responding to any verbal communication, you can adjust your own behaviour. In this way you will demonstrate empathy and offer support when needed.

It is very important to remember that it is impossible to completely understand someone else's feelings, even if we have had a very similar experience ourselves. This is because each of us has a different perception of events. In order to make sense of our experiences we each take on board different elements or factors and link them to existing schema in our memory. Bartlett (1932) speaks of constructive and inferential memory, while Kelly (1955) considers individuals to be like scientists in that we construct an hypothesis then test it out to verify or reject it. On meeting unfamiliar people we may make an assumption about them. Over time as we get to know the person better, we adjust our thoughts or theories.

To summarise so far, caring is a career of complexity and cannot rely on common sense. It is complex because human beings are complex. Every person is a unique individual as a direct result of biology, socialisation, self-perception and ethnicity. Carers need to be sensitive to others and to gain insight into the way another person perceives the world around them in order to be able to assess need, and to work with that person to meet their need.

Groups

Just as all clients are individual, so are staff. All that has been said about working with clients is therefore true when working with a range of care staff. The majority of carers work in groups, but what is meant by group? The Oxford Dictionary defines a group as:

'. . . number of persons or things standing together; number of persons or things belonging or classed together . . .'

The problem with this definition is that it is too vague to be helpful when considered in a caring context. This is a lesson to be learnt when studying health and social care as the dictionary is not always the most appropriate reference when trying to understand the terminology used for sociological and psychological perspectives!

There are perhaps as many different definitions of groups as there are reasons for people coming together to form one! Perhaps one that is relevant to Health and Social Care is that of Sherif and Sherif (1956) when they state:

> A group is a social unit which consists of a number of individuals who stand in (more or less) definite status and role relationships to one another and which possesses a set of values or norms of its own regulating the behaviour of individual members, at least in matters of consequence to the group. (p. 144)

This definition may be applied to Health and Social Care to denote a collection of individuals who come together with the express aim of providing care and support for a particular client group. Each individual has a particular role to play in the provision of care. Group members will have shared values and will establish ways of working together to meet the needs of the clients.

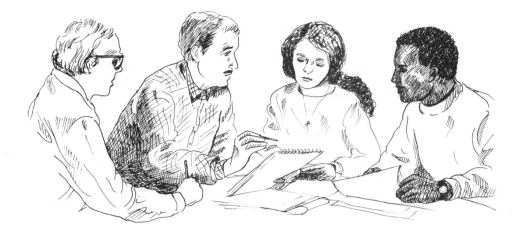

Teamwork

There are numerous texts specifically discussing groups and group processes, in a variety of settings. A list of suggested reading is given at the end of this book which you may find helpful.

Humans are, in the main, social beings preferring to be in the company of others: Rubin and McNeil (1983). Indeed, it has been demonstrated in terms of the development of self-concept that interaction with others plays an important part in the development of an idea of self: Bannister and Agnew (1976).

Reflective activity

Think of the many groups that you belong to: from family to social group, perhaps a religious or ethnic group. What is it that brings the different individuals together?

Psychologists see membership of groups as meeting psychological needs. For example, Freud saw group membership as meeting the need of an adult to replace the family. By this, Freud considered that the need for a leader was the need for a parental figure; the need for group members was equated to the need for siblings.

Other individual needs may be sought in a group, for example, affiliation needs, i.e. to be accepted by others rather than isolated; or the need for power in terms of viewing the support of others as being more effective than working alone. Another need is for information: it is possible to compare one's individual perception of the world with that of others and so confirm it.

Group dynamics

When a collection of individuals come together for a particular purpose, they interact with each other and become dependent on each other in order to complete the task in hand. The processes that the group go through may be seen as being dynamic, i.e. they are active rather than passive, powerful rather than weak, and may constantly change thus drawing the individual members together.

Psychologist Kurt Lewin (1948) is considered to be the father of group dynamics. He viewed human behaviour as being a combination of the individual person's characteristics and the characteristics of the environment. When individuals form a group they bring to that group their own characteristics, which need to be acknowledged and harmonised with the characteristics of others if the group is to function effectively. In other words the individuals have to find ways of supporting each other. They do this by acknowledging individual strengths and weaknesses so that collectively the best use of resources is made to complete the task.

It is important to note that the term 'group dynamics' refers not only to the processes involved in groups but also to the scientific study of groups as well. Both sociologists and psychologists study group dynamics to gain a deeper understanding of the impact on groups of various factors – such as societal factors in the case of sociologists. Psychologists study the impact of emotions and behaviour and individual thought.

Reflective activity

The skills required to be an active group member are many. They draw on how you perceive yourself. Think of an occasion when you joined a new group of people for the first time. It might be the first day at a new school or college, or the first day at a new job. How did you feel? Did anything happen to help you feel welcome or were you feeling quite isolated?

Self-esteem

It helps if you feel confident in yourself, but even so we all feel some apprehension when joining an existing group. Why do you think this is? To answer such a question it is necessary to look once again at the theory of self-concept discussed in Chapter 1.

Another theory to consider is Kelly's Personal Construct Theory (1955). Kelly's theory involves the need to be able to predict in order to control. The need to predict may be used to explain feelings of apprehension when facing a new group of people. If the individual has no prior experience of the members of the group, he/she cannot predict how he/she will be received. This uncertainty may lead to anxiety as one cannot take control of a situation if one is unable to predict the reaction of others. Perhaps there is also uncertainty regarding one's acceptability, i.e. that the need for acceptance and approval by others will be met.

As a member of the existing group it would be important to welcome a new member and to introduce them to the other group members, allowing time for each to give a little information about themselves as an introduction. This shared personal information, however brief, begins to help a new member feel a little more at ease.

Group formation

Tuckman (1965) and Tuckman and Jensen (1977) suggest that when individuals come together for a specific purpose, they pass through a series of five stages.

- **Forming**, the first stage, is perceived as being a time when individuals begin to gain some insight into other people and the tasks in hand. A period of getting to know one another if you like, when opinions are formed about each other, about self in relation to others and their ideas in relation to one's own. This stage is referred to as the forming or orientation stage.

- **Storming**, the second stage, can be quite threatening to some. It is during this stage that individuals may try to press their point of view at the expense of others, which may result in conflict. Some individuals may find the conflict difficult to deal with, so they abstain from the group or make alliances with a few others who hold similar views, resulting in discord and disunity. This storming or conflict stage is unproductive: too many possibly conflicting ideas of how to perform the task in hand will lead to dissatisfaction amongst the members and little will be achieved. Some individuals may even feel marginalised and threatened by others and become uncooperative, leading to the same result.

- **Norming**, the third stage, is when members start to find a common policy. This will clarify the roles and methods by which the group may jointly work to achieve agreed goals. Members of the group will begin to define the values shared by all and define a way of 'doing things', i.e. group culture. Group norms developed through discussion give this stage its name of norming or cohesion, as agreement is reached and a cohesive policy for action developed.

- **Performing**, the fourth stage, sees the group working together to meet the needs of the task in hand by sharing decisions and working together to solve any problems that may arise. Individuals are confident about their own role and accept the role of others in order to achieve the agreed aims. The group are performing well together, hence the name performance or performing stage.

- **Ending**, the fifth and final stage, is an important one, particularly for groups who come together for a limited time. Individuals have become dependent on each other in order to perform the tasks in hand. On completion of tasks the group may be dispersed or re-formed to begin a new task with a different membership in whole or part. Ending a group can be as painful as joining one: the roles change, the motivation to keep the close relationships becomes less and this can be an emotional time.

Reflective activity

Think of a group that you have been in which ended; it could be the group of friends when you leave school, college or work and move on to something else. The role you played in the original group changes and over time you may have found that you had less in common than previously. The group is dissolved or adjourned and there are often mixed emotions at the time which need to be dealt with.

Tuckman's successive-stage theory (1965) is one of several models of group development. Bale's (1965) equilibrium model, for example, perceives the need for group members to keep a balance between achieving the task in hand and improving the quality of relationships and interaction among the group. Sometimes the group will expend more energy on the relationships than on the task and vice versa.

It is important to note that groups may speedily pass from one stage to another or may appear to get stuck at a stage. The group is then deemed to be dysfunctional, or failing to work properly, as little is achieved and individuals become dissatisfied. Indeed in some instances a group appears to regress, or go backwards, and needs time to re-evaluate the situation. The help of an outside 'consultant' may be necessary to enable group members to review the situation objectively. Team-building exercises may also be necessary to help the individuals to begin to build or rebuild relationships and gain some cohesion to enable the group to function.

Teams

Caring usually involves working as part of a team or network in order to meet client need. Many of the factors you may have listed in the exercise at the beginning of this chapter, could apply when working with staff.

Evidence opportunity

You may wish to ask a colleague in your workplace to place your list in rank order from the point of view of working together in a particular care setting. It would again be useful to discuss any differences that may arise, so that you are able to be more effective as a team member.

In care settings a team is a group of people who work together to meet the aims of the establishment, for example, a day nursery providing care for an early years group, or a voluntary organisation which aims to meet the social needs of people with learning difficulties.

There is a view that teams create themselves. Many managers find to their cost that this is not only untrue but dangerous. Another wrong idea is that staff groups are teams. This view is false as it defines neither the quality of the group activity, nor the staff involved in it. A team is more than a group – it is about being clear why you are here. This may be explained in a mission statement held by the establishment. This gives the aim of the establishment, while the collective recognition and agreed task necessary to achieve the aim are the objectives. Much has been written about teams (see John Adair, *Effective Team Building*, 1987), however it is important to emphasise a few points.

Dysfunctional groups

Teams are more powerful than any one leader if their power is used effectively. Team power can bring down an organisation, as some unions did in their struggle for better working conditions. There is a theory that some managers have a lot invested in their teams not working, i.e. being dysfunctional. This makes individuals more reliant on the manager; teams then have less power in the organisation. This serves to maintain the status quo, keep things the same, where change is resisted by the manager. In this context the manager would prefer the teams to argue among themselves rather than with him or her!

In contrast to this, the power of a team can be used to bring down a manager or organisation for destructive purposes. This is where there are one or two strong characters with whom the manager clashes and is unable to challenge. These characters may have been given too much power, and may have decided to use it for their own ends. As a result there may be conflict and damage to the organisation.

Functional group

Alternatively, the team can use its power constructively to empower the manager and themselves to achieve the task more effectively. Action centred leadership has three needs, individual, task and team. If a powerful individual wants their needs met and is not interested in the task or team, they manipulate others towards achieving their own goal. Inevitably there will be casualties and victims.

Leadership

A strong leader needs to challenge this from the beginning and keep it on the agenda, in that every time the team meets this problem is addressed. In this context, the term team means working successfully together, otherwise only a group of individuals exists. A team is a group of staff who are clear about their task, leadership and roles within the group. There is a high degree of trust and openness. Further, the team members are prepared to take risks within the group, i.e. challenge another member of staff without fear of retribution. A team invests a great deal in its maintenance: it looks after and supports each other. (This is explained in further detail on p. 143.)

Evidence opportunity ─────────────────────────────────────

Do you have a team at college or at placement? Observe the way the different individuals go about their work. Take note of the ways individuals interact and support each other in order to achieve group tasks. You will need to undertake this task with sensitivity and may wish to discuss this with your tutor.

Force-field analysis

Problems can often emerge in a team which cannot be resolved despite the expert skill of the leader. A very simple yet effective exercise can be used to unblock or resolve the problem. This exercise is called **force-field analysis**, first described by Kurt Lewin, and is often used in situations where there are forces resisting change. This exercise is also used in counselling and supervision as a way of unblocking and helping people to move on.

Look at the diagram below, and note the restraining forces and driving forces. The restraining forces are all the things which maintain the status quo, i.e. keep the problem or issue constant. The driving forces are the positive things which prompt change and overcome the pressure from the resisting forces.

Force Field Analysis

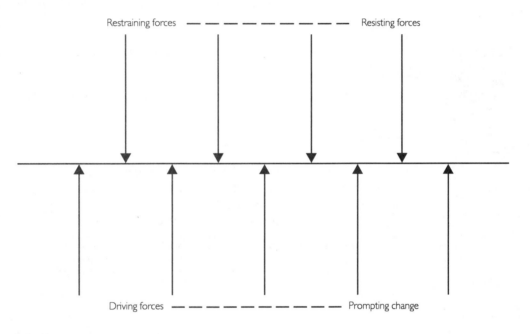

By completing this exercise you will begin to shift the current situation towards the desired position: you prompt change. Each force is identified and examined and action is planned. The theory is simple: you break down the large problem into a series of smaller problems. By tackling each small problem in turn, the whole problem is gradually solved and seems a much more manageable task! In the end the driving forces will have overcome the resisting forces and prompted change.

Evidence opportunity

- Think of a problem, describe the present situation and then describe the desired situation you would like to reach. For example, you have difficulty asking for help with evidence collection for this unit.
- List all the things (resisting forces) which are keeping it a problem.
- Now list all the positive things (driving forces) which will prompt change, i.e. which will get you to seek help with evidence collection.

Work role

It does not matter which client group you eventually work with, you will be expected to work in cooperation with other staff in order to achieve the aims of the establishment. This means that each has to know their own duties and responsibilities, and how those link with the work of others. It is also important to check that your understanding of your role and responsibilities is the same as that of the manager.

A good starting point will be the job description provided for your role. This should give details of the duties and responsibilities you are expected to undertake, and will outline the line management of your role, i.e. what you are responsible for and whom you are responsible to.

Failure to have a clear understanding of what is expected of you can lead to confusion, stress and demotivation. There is an increased risk of conflict with other staff when people feel threatened, complaining that their work is being 'taken over' by others, so they may become uncooperative.

Reflective activity

Think of a time when you have been asked to do something without being given clear guidelines. Can you remember what you did and how you felt? How did other people react to you at the time?

Network

Where a group of people working together have to liaise frequently with other professionals from outside the unit to meet client need, then it is referred to as a network (Hey, 1979), e.g. a hospital ward. Webb and Hobdell (1980) use a useful analogy of sport to demonstrate the difference between a team and a network (see Table 5.1).

Table 5.1 **Sports analogies for teams and networks**

	Team ◄—————————————————————————► Network		
Unit type	Football team	Tennis team	Athletics team
Overall objectives	To win matches	To win matches	To win matches
Specific objectives	Together to score goals Together to defend own goal	To win own match amongst several	To win specific events which are very different from each other
Basic tasks and skills required	Ball control, common to all, marginal specialisation, interchangeability possible	Common (to play tennis!) but specialist in singles/doubles	Most skills unique to each event or task
Amount of face to face work in unit	All work carried out together – feedback and support given live	Little or no work is face to face, feedback and support tailored to individual needs	Little or no work face to face – general collegiate feedback across members not possible in specific terms
Typical social service units	'Intake' team of social workers. Small family group home. House Unit in CHE. Specialist 'child in care' team. Patch team	Area social work team Group of Residential advisors Team of long-term case workers	Area Social Services team (SWs, HHOs, IT workers, OTs etc.) Large CHE Multi-disciplinary staff of hospital ward

Reflective activity

- Think about your own placement or work setting; using the sporting analogy above, are you working in a team or network? Supervision will be essential in order to ensure the quality of care provided by each staff member contributes to the achievement of the overall aim of the unit, whichever model applies.
- Think about a hospital ward; the aim is to diagnose and treat an individual who is ill, e.g. with appendicitis. There will be a team of nurses who work shifts to care for the individual, yet that team must liaise with other professionals to help restore the person's health.

The network of others will include the surgeon, anaesthetist, porters, theatre nursing staff, staff in the laboratories where blood samples are analysed, to name but a few. Each needs to link with the nursing team to assist this person before, during and after his/her appendix is removed. All those working in this network aim to return the individual to full health as speedily as possible through their cooperative efforts.

Evidence opportunity

See if you can give a further example of a network by reviewing a Social Work or Social Care work setting. You may wish to use this as possible evidence by analysing the group in terms of the management style it adopts.

It has been stated that for a group to function, the individual members need to be aware of their particular role within the general framework. Hare (1976), for example, shows the need for members to recognise the requirement for a leader and that others will then follow that lead. In any given group interaction individuals will adopt specific roles in order to assist the group to function.

During any one day each individual subtly alters the way they interact with others by adapting their behaviour to meet their perception of the expectation of others.

Reflective activity

- Think of the way you interact with an older member of the family, a senior person at work, a close friend, a younger person. Each of those people will have a schema which helps them to determine the way you will to behave when interacting with them – you therefore adapt your behaviour to meet that perception as closely as possible.
- To gain a better insight, think of how you expect a doctor to behave in a surgery or a lecturer in college. If these people behave very differently to the way we expect, we think of their behaviour as abnormal since it does not conform with our preconceived ideas of the way a person in that position or role should behave. We stereotype doctors, expecting them to behave in similar ways when providing care and attention.

Roles within groups

Individuals take on a variety of roles when working in groups. The roles fall into two distinct categories of task, as suggested by Benne and Sheats (1948), for example, an information seeking role and socio-emotional or maintenance roles, e.g. an encourager who nods in agreement and smiles to offer support to an individual during a meeting.

Evidence opportunity

Arrange to sit in on a staff group meeting at your workplace. (A group of five or six is ideal. You will need to negotiate this with staff to explain what you are doing and why.) Carefully observe what goes on in terms of the roles that different group members adopt. You may record this using a sociogram (see the diagram below).

Sociograms

Sociograms are a way of pictorially recording interaction between members of a group. Draw a box or circle to represent each group member to show the position of each member in relation to the others. Give each person a code and draw an arrow from that person to the person or persons they are speaking to on each occasion they make a contribution. If the individual is addressing their remarks to all members, then draw the arrow to the centre of the group.

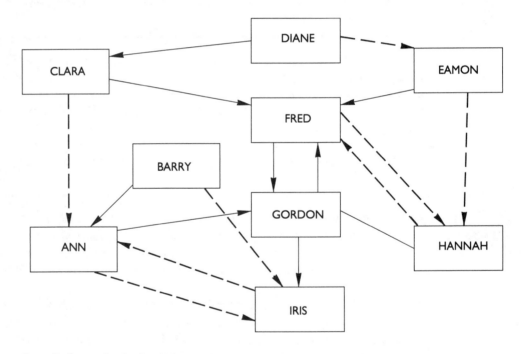

Example of a completed sociogram

You will need to analyse your findings to note the contributions of the different members and you may notice that some do not contribute to the group but perhaps form a sub-group, addressing their comments to one other person only. What effect did this sub-group have on the functioning of the whole group?

Evidence opportunity

Look at the sociogram given as an example; what can you learn from this about the roles that the individual members took? Did a sub-group emerge and was there an apparent leader?

It takes time to be able to complete sociograms successfully; it comes with practice and you may find it easier to video a group meeting so that you can replay it as often as you like! (Do gain permission before attempting to do this.) Perhaps a role play of a meeting with friends will be helpful. You will need to accustom people to the presence of the camera or you may find that people are too self-conscious to behave normally!

Individuals joining a group will initially be unsure about the possible role they will play in order to complete the task. As the group settles and begins to function then individual roles within the general scheme of things are clarified. Stress and confusion will occur if the particular role expected of one person is unclear. Perhaps a new post is created and the person given that post has no idea what is expected of them, and because it is new there is no one to refer to in order to gain clarification – this is termed 'role ambiguity'. The group will need to assist the individual to outline their perception of the parameters of the new post so that the individual can be confident to proceed.

Role conflict arises when there are differing demands made on the same individual so that they are unsure what is expected of them.

Reflective activity

Imagine that you are working in a residential setting as a carer. Due to illness you are short staffed and are having to be carer, cook and manager. Each role has differing demands on your time and the conflict occurs when you are prioritising tasks to ensure a quality service is maintained.

Similarly you may find that being a student causes a role conflict between that of student and that of partner or friend. If your student role means that studies and/or work experience leaves limited time to meet the demands made by your partner or friend, this may lead to feelings of guilt and it will take time to work through to a compromise.

The skills required to be an effective group member are many. It may be useful to review the work of Carl Rogers (1961) who speaks of accepting self and others, of demonstrating positive regard. This means that we build relationships with others based on trust by recognising each as an individual with the right to respect, for example, and by working with colleagues and clients in a supportive manner, accepting them as they are without making judgements.

To build a relationship with others in a group means being prepared to listen to another point of view and to share ideas, being willing to compromise, being realistic about oneself. All of these depend on the way each person perceives themselves in terms of a positive self-concept. If an individual has low self-esteem then it is very much harder to feel able to express an opinion, particularly if that opinion differs from the one held by the majority, i.e. it is difficult to be assertive.

Success in working with others comes about by clear communication and support of each other in order to achieve previously agreed aims or goals (Douglas, 1991). When each member is made to feel valued in their role, then they gain a measure of satisfaction even in a very demanding role. This helps to maintain motivation and acts to stimulate other members. This in turn leads to a functional team working in general harmony to achieve the aim of the group.

Characteristics of a good group member

What characteristics make for an effective group member?

- An individual who is willing to listen and effectively communicate with others to share knowledge and experience.
- An individual who is willing to be flexible and responsible enough to take on a particular role.
- An individual who is conscientious and reliable, a creative thinker and active problem solver.
- An individual who is able to work in cooperation with others but has initiative and can work within the boundaries of the group.
- An individual who is able to acknowledge their own skills and remain realistic regarding their limitations, willing to seek advice and support when necessary.

The list is not exhaustive but goes some way to show the many facets of working in groups. You should add any others that come to mind. Each of the above outlines the case for an individual to be self-aware, self-confident and assertive: self-aware in recognising and acknowledging one's own strengths and weaknesses, self-confident in having a positive self-image, and assertive enough to be able to voice an opinion without resorting to aggression when a difference of opinion arises.

Reflective activity

Imagine that you have recently been employed as a care worker in a residential unit for a group of adults with learning disabilities. The unit has two day shifts at the weekend when most of the residents are at home. On your first day you are placed with a member of staff who has been in the post for some years. He seems slightly annoyed to have the task of instructing you and is brusque (sharp) in his manner as he gives instructions but no explanations to you. He does not introduce you to any residents or staff and seems to expect you to follow his movements quickly as he goes about his duties.

You watch other staff during the day and notice that each seems to work in their own way. You notice that one person is never invited to join the others and comments are made about her when she leaves the room. There are constant remarks about the workload and poor resources are often quoted as the reason why little stimulation is available for the residents. Staff seem quite apathetic despite their apparent concern for the residents.

To gain some insight into this scenario, it is important to think again about the reasons why people commit themselves to a particular career. If you can accept that people are motivated to work to gain personal satisfaction and fulfilment, then it is important to look at the means of achieving that fulfilment.

Much depends on the quality of the management in that a manager must ensure that the member of staff has the knowledge and skill to undertake the role allocated to them.

Failure to do that leads to demotivation, frustration and stress for the individual. The staff team in this imagined example seem to have little support from management who appear to expect staff to do more without explaining the reasons. Lack of communication between staff and managers may well be an issue here. Management issues will be explored in detail in the following chapter.

Secondly it is important that staff receive feedback on their performance and are told when a job is done well. Often staff face criticism for errors and successful work goes unrecognised! Think how you felt last time someone told you that you had done something well. Did you find that it encouraged you to continue? Supervision of staff would go some way towards demonstrating the importance of each person and giving encouragement at a time of stress for all.

Morale in this establishment is obviously low, and staff appear to be demotivated, completing only tasks they see to be essential. The member of staff you were placed with perhaps felt that you were just another worry to add to his load. Resourcing is an issue in the 1990s but is it being used as an excuse for inaction? What about the person being isolated by the rest of the group? What about you in the scenario – how might assertiveness help to improve the quality of your experience?

Management will need to work to review the situation as speedily as possible. Work is needed to assess each individual need and to build the staff group into a team. Failure to do so will lead to further lowering of morale and increased stress levels among the staff. High stress among staff will result in a poor service to the residents and possibly high levels of staff illness, resulting in yet more change for the residents to cope with. According to Tuckman's theory of group development, this group may be seen as in the storming stage. See what you think and compare this theory with the detail in the following chapter.

Care staff have responsibilities in a group setting but need the support of management while the individual develops personally and professionally. The support available to care staff working within a group will be addressed in the following chapter dealing with management issues.

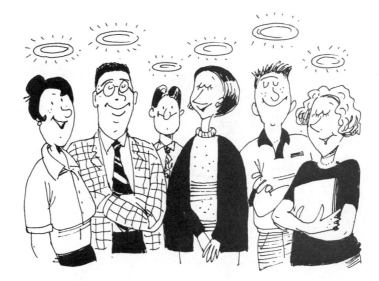

Stereotype of carers

6 Management of care settings

What is covered in this chapter

- What is management?
- Why study management?
- Management in residential care
- Skills of management
- Supervision
- Coping with stress
- Managing change
- Equal opportunities in management

What is management?

Management is a term often bandied about to mean many things. It is this lack of clarity that often creates mystique about a subject which everyone has something to say about yet little understanding of its true nature. When things go wrong management is blamed; when staff don't get a pay rise or the promotion they were seeking, again management is blamed; and when a customer wants to complain it is somehow management's responsibility. But who is or are the management?

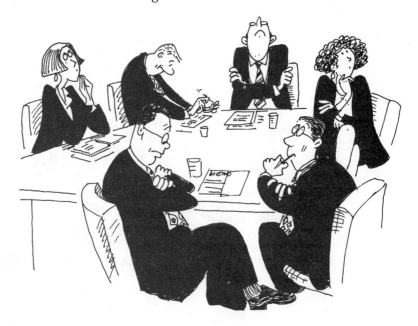

Who are the management?

There are probably as many terms to define management as there are people practising it. There are two definitions which may be found particularly useful. The first definition is designed to give focus and meaning to management:

> **To manage human resource potential by maximising individual growth output;**

and the second is taken from John Harvey-Jones, the well known ex-chairman of ICI:

> **Management in particular is not about the preservation of the status quo, it is about maintaining the highest rate of change that the organisation and the people within it can stand. (1990, p. 14)**

In both these definitions roles and people are excluded. Management is about a process and it is this process that the definitions attempt to define. Every person filling a role manages something at some time; performing these roles does not always result in being called a manager. Everyone manages something even if it is only their time.

You will see from the first definition that management is about using your resources well. The best resources a **care setting** has are the people that work within it. Management is about ensuring that staff are happy, well motivated and give their maximum to the job. If the staff are well looked after and in return work harder, this is more likely to result in greater productivity for the organisation.

The second definition (which is presently being given greater attention) looks at the amount of change an organisation can stand. You might have heard, through the media, of difficulties that this country has been experiencing over the years. One of the reasons given is that the amount of change we are going through is too fast for the country to cope with. For example, in the field of caring, within a year three major pieces of legislation were brought into force:

- Children Act 1989
- Community Care Act 1990
- Juvenile Justice Act 1991.

These new Acts created difficulties for local authorities because despite the legislation being phased in over several years, the resource implications and structural problems were immense; consequently many authorities could not cope. Many social services departments reorganised, changing people's jobs overnight. People had to learn new skills and new roles which they had not been prepared for. Further, in the area of Community Care, services were split into what is known as 'purchaser' and 'provider' roles. Purchaser services assess, negotiate and organise services, whereas providers deliver them.

This is a totally new concept which will take many years to integrate fully into existing ways of working. Moreover the people who are responsible for carrying out such new roles will need years to learn how the details of such roles will work. It means people have to learn new skills, adopt different attitudes and acquire different knowledge. Much of this was not anticipated by the government. Consequently many staff may leave the profession because they cannot cope with the stress caused by this change. The clients/customers/purchasers suffer as there may be a shortage of staff to provide them with the services needed.

Change is crucially important and is an area which all employees must understand. John Harvey-Jones's quote refers to initiating change, as this keeps you ahead of the market; change is needed in order to survive. During the recession of the early nineties many companies directed their energies into maintaining the status quo instead of changing it, i.e. keeping things the way they have always been, such as retaining traditions which have been handed down in the family for generations, which may be honourable but does not make managerial sense. What happens is that more efficient companies come along who successfully predict the change in consumer need, thus leaving their competitors out in the cold.

During the era of change in the 1980s the concept of 'individualism' was introduced and caring took on a different notion which was based on what John Harvey-Jones calls a new ethic – the strongest organisations will survive. But perhaps a part of that survival took on board a new cultural morality, where standards that used to be acceptable are no longer, as portrayed in the following quote from Charles Handy:

> In a world of individualism the dominant ethic can so easily become 'What harms no one is OK', or 'What the others do and get away with has to be alright', or even 'If no one knows then you're fine.' (1989, p. 208)

Elderly people who need residential care now have a choice in where they want to live. No longer can a local authority place all its clients in one place. If their residential home is not up to standard they may be forced to close it for lack of referrals. They need to compete. Everyone in the private, voluntary and public sectors will be competing for business. For example, an old style residential care home manager in the public sector now requires business skills in marketing as they have to offer something in competition with private homes. Yet so often they are not given the skills and fail badly. Business sense is of great importance.

Everyone at work manages, but do they all manage well? Management is about using your existing resources well, by getting the best out of what you have and directing energy towards maintaining constant change. Those people who do not want to change may have to leave because conflict for them will probably become unbearable. Remember, if you are not changing you are not moving; if you are not moving you stand still and because nothing stands still in business you go backwards, and thus fail.

Reflective activity

Spend a few minutes to create your own definition of management and see how it compares with the task of the manager at the end of this chapter.

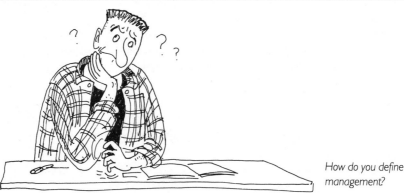

How do you define management?

Why study management?

In business, studying management is necessary in order to understand the importance of using your resources well and ensuring that they are directed towards the right market-place. It therefore seems relevant that management should be an essential element of any curriculum. In the care sector the greatest resource is the people within it, which means you. You are so valuable and such an asset that unless you are maintained and cared for, you will fade like an old painting which has been left in the loft and forgotten. In management there are many people whose goal and ambition is primarily to put the client first, themselves second and the staff team third. Management is also about survival, because if you don't survive, you are not able to reap the rewards you may have been working so hard for.

Your first responsibility as a student worker or manager is to yourself. You come first when the chips are down. If you do not survive then you have nothing left to offer your clients. Do not feel guilty about this. Anyone who speaks otherwise may be fooling themselves. Your second responsibility is to your team, and for managers it is to their staff – without staff and teams there may be nothing to offer the client as they are the greatest resource assets available. After these, priorities should then be directed towards the clients themselves.

When staff are under pressure it is then that mistakes are made. If staff are not in a healthy state because they have been working under stress for too long or without guidance or support, then they are dangerous to themselves and others. Staff under extreme stress and who are without support or supervision are unpredictable and more likely to react in a way that they would not normally. They may behave unprofessionally towards the client. The same can be said for any relationship and interaction which goes on within the context of stress. If you are left unsupported in your family and have to cope with acute levels of pressure you may crack up. In a professional role you could lose your job and your career.

It is essential in studying management to know why things go wrong, why it is that your team keep arguing and never reach a decision, or why one particular member always attempts to sabotage meetings. If you are working with groups in a daily situation you will need to know how groups and teams function. It is also important to know how to receive and give support, as a lack of support can lead to a failure to care for others.

You also need to know what your role is and what is expected of you. This can often be found in what is called a **job specification** which highlights all the tasks, essential or otherwise, that are important to the job. When you start in any new job there should be a period of induction which, if nothing else, clarifies your role so that you are clear about what you are trying to achieve. A good section on induction can be found in Terry Scraggs, *Managing to Care* (1993).

Management in residential care

Before 1984 residential homes had little independent inspection or monitoring, some say none at all. Consequently the type of care was often poor. For example, in the private sector good care may sometimes have been sacrificed for the need to make profits. Unqualified and low paid care assistants were taken on to undertake the main tasks of caring. There was often no system of ensuring someone's suitability for working with the elderly. For example, a person with a criminal record for abuse could be employed. However the local authority sector fared no better, and cutbacks often forced local authorities to compromise levels of care in areas where there was least public pressure, e.g. the elderly. In 1984 legislation was passed forcing local authorities to inspect all residential homes (although not their own); this was called the Registered Homes Act 1984. Most of this Act was founded on the work done by the Centre for Policy on Ageing in their publication *Home Life* (1984) and it was envisaged that the 218 recommendations would be taken up.

Home Life did little to improve standards in real terms and government inquiries led to tighter legislation. With the publication of the Wagner Report (1988) on residential care and the Community Care legislation in 1991, independent inspection units were set up to monitor and set standards of care for all residential homes including local authority homes. It is worth reading the Health Department's guidance on residential homes for the elderly, mentally ill and disabled, which sets the standards managers must adhere to.

Management in residential homes is now very different to the way it was, in that the role of the manager has changed. There is new guidance, and laws setting new standards and targets which a manager must achieve. There is a competitive climate where customers have to be attracted to a residential home. There is also the task of having to juggle with budgets. All in all management is a very complex task.

Delegation

Managers today have to be all things to all people and many of them have not been trained or given the skills to cope with this new challenge. For example, to delegate might appear to be an easy solution. Yet many managers cannot because they do not have anyone to delegate to. Most of their staff may be unqualified and certainly have not had the specialised training to cope with the new demands being made of them. This is the task for the new manager. They need to be able to demonstrate how to do the job, to act as a role model, yet be able to start a programme of training to ensure that in the near future there will be people to delegate to. This broad approach is essential because no manager would be able to cope with a massive workload for any sustained length of time.

Supervision

In their new role managers must also ensure staff receive adequate supervision as laid down in statutory guidance. Again this takes planning and time. Much of the time and energy previously spent in residential care went on the direct care of the client, for example, washing, feeding, clothing, cooking, cleaning, talking to them, advising them, etc. Now staff often have to perform at a more professional level (e.g. within the new framework of an NVQ value base); they will require support if they are to give support. Managers are responsible for providing an empowering and supportive environment for their staff.

Training

Staff now have to attend training courses (maybe for some it will be their first time), yet to achieve this goal requires some sophisticated planning with the staff rota. All care settings have a rota system of staff working shifts. In most homes the staff and client ratio cannot be altered to allow staff time off to attend training. Training has to be organised within existing resources. If you speak to many managers and ask them about their role they will often explain their experience is of having to be like a magician – sometimes they are expected to perform miracles.

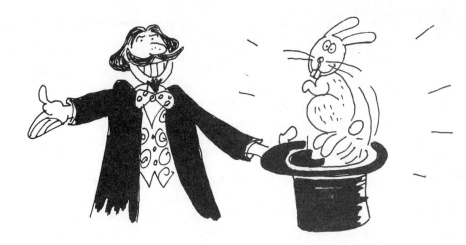

A manager is thought by some to be a magician!

Introducing change

Many people who have worked in the care system for a substantial number of years see their work as a vocation and they resist changes. They might see the way they have always removed people from their beds in the morning in an almost military fashion as being efficient and effective. 'I've done it like that for years and no one has ever complained.' Yet there was no mechanism to complain; now in law, there is a complaints procedure which all homes must publish and make available to all their users and anyone with an interest.

A manager who forces change on such people overnight is heading for trouble. If you bash someone over the head hard enough or for long enough they might eventually give up, and in the case of a care worker they might eventually leave. But if this is a manager's objective, they may end up with no staff. The balance is in trying to achieve a compromise. Implement change slowly and with everyone's involvement at every stage.

It is a tricky business trying to keep a happy staff team, yet a happy staff team means a happy care setting. Whatever a manager decides will inevitably not please everyone. It helps sometimes if staff can have insight into a manager's job, so that they are then in a better position to empathise. It is also the team's responsibility to support the manager – support must never be just one way. A manager who feels insecure and hangs on to the controls tightly, never sharing information or delegating, may cause discontent amongst the team. The team will resent the lack of trust given to them. Any situation where the facts are not disclosed opens itself up to speculation. A lack of staff understanding may create an anti-management culture which becomes destructive to the management of the care setting.

Evidence opportunity

If you work in a team on placement or in your studies, try to identify the roles each member plays and who leads. Try to imagine where you fit in the team.

Skills of management

Any student of management requires some understanding of its theory base. However, it would be impossible in this short text to cover all the various theories which could help inform our understanding of what management is about. A good synopsis of management theory can be found in Veronica Coulshed's work *Management in Social Work* (1992), in particular, Chapters 1 and 2.

Some of the areas essential to good management are referred to here with suggested reading for further information.

Planning

Good planning will be seen as the cornerstone of all successful organisations. What do we mean by planning? Firstly most organisations are clear about what they are for. They have what is known as a **mission statement**. This is a statement of purpose, a sort of aim which the organisation intends to achieve coupled with its belief or value base. For example, a mission statement of an organisation providing residential care homes might say something like the following:

> All residents will be treated equally, with respect and dignity. The home will provide these people with a caring environment that enables its residents to live individually as well as happily together.

It is from this statement of purpose (mission statement) that all other planning will be made.
- Operational planning is the day to day management of running the home; what things need to be considered, decided upon and organised – anything from organising the rota to bulk ordering of the food.
- Strategic planning is the more long-term planning, which is about direction, where we are going, and might include discussions on marketing, or extending the service currently being offered.

Strategic planning encompasses the long-term goals which often include a five year plan. For example, a strategic plan might aim to explore the difficulty that exists in attracting black residents to come and live in a multicultural setting. It may require some soul searching to establish the difficulties, and then implementation of necessary changes in order to attract and encourage black people to live there.

Management by objectives

Another aspect of planning is to ensure you have the right objectives in place before you start. This is known as **Management by Objectives** (MBO) from the work of Peter Drucker in 1954 (Glaser, 1987). MBO is really a 'systems approach' to planning. It is about linking all the employees' individual plans to the overall organisational plan (which might be the mission statement). Imagine a difficult task, say a female care assistant dressing an elderly man who makes sexual advances to female staff. There is no male assistant available to help. You need to sit down with the entire staff team and plan together. You need to consider the organisation's goal of what it wants to achieve (the mission statement), such as emphasising the individuality of residents, yet staff needs include not wanting to be sexually assaulted! A strategy needs to be devised and tested. The outcome of the plan is evaluated by the staff and changes are made. It is a process of:

→ INPUT – ACTIVITIES – OUTPUT →

This is a very simplified explanation. However 'Input – Activities – Output' is often used successfully in many areas of management and not just problem solving. Recently it has been linked with staff appraisal. Each year staff have the quality of their work assessed. Management by Objectives is worked out for the following year and evaluated at the end of that year. Many companies, education and social services use the concept of performance related pay. Staff must reach certain targets worked out by objectives to achieve their bonus or percentage of pay. There is much argument about this approach, especially in education where performance is linked to end results, i.e. the exams children passed or whether they can read at the age of seven. Many educators would say you cannot measure progress by the end result. It is the process of getting there which is more important, i.e. whether the young person experienced the time learning at school as a positive experience or not.

Leadership

This is such an enormous area that we can only make brief reference to it here. There are many theories and styles of leadership. Leadership in the care sector is an extremely important subject. All organisations, groups and teams need leadership. Is leadership about being in charge of people? It could be, but more often it is about getting the best from your team in a given situation they are faced with. The leader may change depending on the situation being faced. For example, in a crisis a particular member of staff may be excellent in taking charge and leading everyone while in a different situation someone else would be more appropriate.

This is known as **Situational Leadership Theory**. You select the right style for the task. This assumes there is no one best style. The manager develops the behaviour of the team to work for him/her in adapting to meet the demands of their own unique situation.

Another form of leadership equally important and effective in the care setting derives from John Adair's model known as **Action Centred Leadership** (1979). He refers to the topic of needs by stating that there are three basic needs a manager must meet. Illustrated in the diagram on p. 144, they are:
- the needs of the team
- the needs of the individuals in the team
- the needs of the task (the job they are there for).

When things go wrong it is often because there is an imbalance, i.e. only individual or task needs are being met. The team suffers and as a result do not see themselves as a group.

Managers have to balance their time and energy into the three areas – this is known as maintenance. If too much energy is devoted to one person, it may be at the cost of one of the other needs. The skill is in being able to meet all three needs. Of course this is an impossible task to achieve all the time. If a member of staff is in a crisis then of course a lot of effort might go into meeting their needs. This would only be temporary as it could not be sustained for too long without damaging the team or task needs. An effective manager would use the team to support an individual while gaining support to cover their work so the task needs do not suffer. In reality this is extremely difficult as there are many other complicating factors which often get in the way. For example, some staff are not prepared

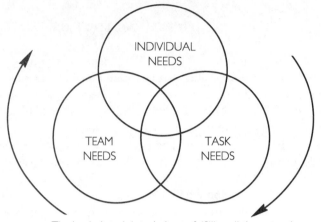

The leader's task is to balance fulfilling all three needs

Action centred leadership

to compromise: they want all of their needs met all of the time and when the manager fails to achieve this the team is blamed and conflict follows.

There are well known styles of leadership developed from the 1930s' classification:

- Autocratic (dictatorial)
- Democratic (following a majority opinion)
- Laissez faire (taking a non-directive role and allowing things to sort themselves out).

All of these have their place in a given situation. Most care worker managers would admit to preferring the democratic style as it sits nicely with the principles of social care in empowering and respecting staff. This is an illusion because each of the other styles are as essential and legitimate. If you think back to your school days, maybe you had a head teacher who ruled like a tyrant; this is clearly demoralising to staff and is not effective. However, if a resident is being abused and staff are covering up for their colleague because they do not want to report them, such leadership may be crucial in protecting the client (autocratic). The manager must sometimes make unilateral or one-sided decisions.

In a different situation where there is not the urgency to respond, then a discussion may involve everyone in making a decision (democratic). In other situations it may be appropriate to sit back and allow your staff to experience responsibility and get on with it (laissez faire). Either way they all have their place in management.

Decision making

This comes easily for some but for others it is one of the most difficult functions for the manager. Much is written about decision making (see Polras, 1989). There are a few basic principles. Where possible no decision should be made on your own, since it is far better to involve others so that responsibility for the consequences of the decision can be shared. Also, people are more likely to go along with a decision that they have been party to. Sometimes, however, a manager has to make a decision on their own and it may be an unpopular one, so it is essential that they make the decision decisively in order that the team should feel confident that they will see it through.

In making decisions there is nothing worse than passing the buck and forcing someone else to take the decision. If this happens to you don't accept responsibility unless it is part of your job role. Going along with weak management is no excuse if you fail later. When making decisions it is best to have all the facts before you so that your judgement is

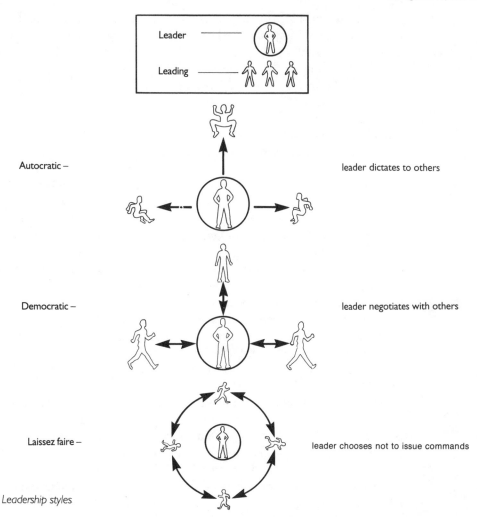

Leadership styles

informed as well as possible. Admitting a bad decision is far better than trying to opt out or being defensive and blaming others at a later stage.

Evidence opportunity

In looking at the skills of planning, leadership and decision making spend some time over the next week observing your manager – or training manager. Do they plan well and lead effectively? What style do they use? Do they delegate or make decisive decisions? Write your observations down and assess how effective you believe them to be. What can you learn from this?

Supervision

In all work in the caring sector good quality supervision is essential. It is so important that without it you cannot develop adequately. With the stresses and strains of care work supervision becomes one of the first things to be dropped when time is short. Supervision has often been seen as a luxury, a good idea if there was time. Yet to some writers it encompasses everything we do in the workplace. Tony Scott and Chris Payne (1982) refer to this as 'Supervision . . . is a process that is integral to the working life of every operational unit.' Supervision is not just about sitting having a chat on a one to one basis and talking nice pleasantries.

There are many models of good supervision; for example, in Gerard Egan's *Skilled Helper* a useful model is given. Egan's model talks about a systematic approach working through three stages. These are:

- looking at the problem
- identifying the problem
- working towards resolution of the problem.

So often there is not the time to be able to do this when immediate action is urgently required. It is important to view a few models and choose the best fit for your situation and skills. No model will cover all situations like leadership – the skill is in the adaptability and transferability of knowledge and skills from one situation to another.

It is important to read and understand something about the theory of supervision not only because one day you might be supervising, but also more importantly so that you can identify good supervision and demand it from your manager and training manager when necessary. There are many methods for achieving good supervision.

- Individual supervision is one of the most common. Usually the manager sees the individual once a week (more often once a month).
- Group supervision is very effective in coaching, using other people's good or bad practice for the team to learn from.
- Peer supervision is where members of the same team take responsibility for each other.

Sometimes an outside consultant is brought in to work with the team or individuals. This is a good idea as it can bring freshness to difficult situations which cannot be resolved within the organisation. A sense of detachment is sometimes all that is needed. Detachment can easily be achieved by bringing someone in from outside who does not necessarily have to have expert knowledge of your client/customer group. Supervision can be used in various forms in addition to using different models.

But what is supervision? Supervision is about three important elements:

- Making the supervisee **accountable** for their tasks. Are they doing and achieving what they should be? Are they doing the job well enough?
- Secondly, it is about **training** so that the individual has an opportunity to learn new skills and knowledge.
- Lastly and more importantly, it is about **personal growth and development**. This is the area which often encroaches on one's personal life.

By using this model the supervisor can ensure that the task, training and personal growth needs are covered. Supervision which is all about tasks (beating someone with a stick to get the job done) will rapidly demotivate staff. Equally, if it is all about personal growth (giving lots of support) the task never gets done and frustration creeps in. There must be a balance between all three, which requires skill and experience and does take some time to achieve. However if you are new to supervision it is important that you are given the opportunity to practise these skills, provided you yourself are being properly supervised to ensure you are gaining the right coaching and support.

Reflective activity

How able are you to share on a personal level things about yourself with your supervisor, tutor or training manager? How does this benefit you?

Good supervision has a high degree of trust and openness. The roles and rules are clear. People know why they are there and what the boundaries are. For example, it is essential that the boundary of confidentiality is clear. This is an important issue which, for some, might limit their disclosure of personal problems affecting work. Good supervision will display some of the following elements:

- Confrontation (facing up to real issues)
- Conflict (being open and supportive about different views)
- Problem solving (defining and resolving the problem)
- Quality feedback on performance (being accountable)
- Appraisal or assessment of work activities (feedback)
- Active listening (reflection)
- Supportive behaviour (warmth, understanding and sincerity)
- Consistency (maintaining good standards)
- Action planning (organising tasks around time constraints)
- Making decisions (taking responsibility)
- Prioritising (organising oneself to make the right decisions)
- Delegating (letting go of responsibility appropriately)
- Learning (personal and professional development)
- Constructive criticism (taking risks for high gain)
- Humour (being real).

Reflective activity

Does your supervision or tutored work include any of these and to what extent?

People need to know that they are doing well. Often good supervision is linked to staff assessment or self-appraisal. Once a year staff are seen by their managers and spend a few hours appraising their work over the year and setting targets for the coming year (depending on the system of appraisal being used). Supervision should be recorded so that if there are disagreements they can be easily checked. One by one staff work through the targets set by the annual appraisal.

Another point often avoided in supervision, but essential if you belong to a minority group, is issues of race, gender, sexuality, disability, etc. If your manager is a man and you are a woman there will be issues of gender despite how aware your supervisor may be of gender differences and using the right language, etc. Consequently there will be some issues a manager cannot empathise with. This is inevitable and should not be seen as a weakness. The issue should be put on the agenda so that it can be referred to in an open and unguarded way. The same will apply if you are black and your manager is white. The facts will always be different and personal to the individual, but what remains the same is the necessity to bring the issue out into the open. For example, if you are white and being supervised by a black manager some issues may be different in terms of power, but there still remain issues of race which warrant addressing or at least acknowledging.

Reflective activity

Spend a few minutes reflecting on this. Would you agree?

Lastly, supervision is not one way, it is a two-way learning process in an interaction which is dynamic, active and developmental. The supervisor has as much to learn as the supervisee and therefore having this attitude can help make supervision successful.

Evidence opportunity

What qualities, skills, etc. do you have which your supervisor can learn from? Make a list.

Coping with stress

Being able to cope with stress is essential to all of us. We all need stress to help us survive but like all things which are good for us too much stress is bad. In the caring profession one is entering a very stress orientated environment, not so much because of the clients and the difficult situations being confronted daily, but because the great pressures being placed on workers in today's climate of financial cutbacks often take their toll. Staff are having to take on more work with less resources in a climate where public pressure and scrutiny is at its peak. In child protection or in residential social work we hear of cases where staff are in fear of confronting teenage boys who are out of control in case they make allegations of improper conduct against them. There was a case where a mother smacked her child which resulted in the mother being reported to the police and later charged with assault (*The Observer*, 22 August 1993). Such a shift in power has resulted in a rise in anxiety for those involved in caring for vulnerable young people. This could have been made worse by the Children Act 1989 which intentionally gave more rights and protection to children but failed to help children or carers cope with this sudden shift in power.

However there is no easy answer to relieving stress as what is one person's cure is another's stressor. It is essential that you build yourself a first aid survival kit before you start in the profession.

Evidence opportunity

Do you know what makes you stressed, how you can recognise it and what do you do to relieve it? Check Chapter 4 if you have not yet done so.

Wagner (1988) talks about residential care and the amount of particular stress this causes to staff and how organisations must respond to this with regular supervision. In a team which is functioning well a good deal of support can be offered to help the staff under stress. In supervision, stress can be identified and dealt with. But if supervision does not exist then there could be a problem, especially if the person is isolated with no outside system of support.

When people become too stressed over a prolonged period of time their body cannot cope and they become ill as the only way of forcing them to stop before they completely break down. Stress related illnesses are legitimate illnesses but are often seen negatively. Stereotyped images are projected about stress causing further damage to people who have stress related problems. Staff suffering from such illness might be viewed as not being able to cope with the job and therefore it is felt that they should not be doing it. In one sense this is true yet it would also be true for anyone attempting to work under such pressure, even if they have not succumbed to stress related illness. People do not become ill through stress lightly. Yet it is still not recognised to the same extent as physical illness. Mental illness which results from stress is often viewed in the workplace as a weakness in the character of the person, rather than a weakness in the organisation for allowing someone to work under such conditions.

If you are relieving stress through what might be seen as negative reactions, for example, drinking heavily, becoming violent, taking drugs and becoming dependent on them, running away, developing abnormal behaviour patterns such as neurotic behaviour, etc., then you need help because your body is taking a double blow, firstly from the original stressor which remains constant, and secondly from the new stressor disguised as a miracle cure, e.g. alcohol. Above all else you should never try to become a hero and sail through your problems in the hope of curing them en route. The residents or clients are often at the receiving end of your own personal disaster, therefore it is more professional and beneficial to your own health to exit while you can and seek the right help, and then come back refreshed. Often people are then in a position to be able to use their experience positively by helping others who are experiencing similar problems. This gives them a more empathetic perspective.

Evidence opportunity

Over the next week watch your colleagues and observe what behaviour they use to exhibit stress. How can you identify it? What do they do to cope? Do they have a first aid survival kit?

Managing change

The concept of change is a new area in management which we are only now beginning to come to terms with, although change has always been taking place. Forty years ago it was easier to predict the next ten years ahead. People who had jobs expected to keep them until they retired, and often jobs would be handed down from father to son, especially in for example, the mining industry. At present it is difficult to predict more than a month in advance, not only because technology is changing so fast that we cannot keep up with it, but also because of the way financial resources have dominated the workplace. Change is occurring more rapidly since industry must respond more immediately to the way the market is moving if it wants to remain in profit. Sometimes situations move quickly without warning. Ten years ago most people in the caring sector would not have predicted that the majority of their jobs would be privatised and the business culture of today would be so influential. Instead of training in counselling distressed clients it is financial accountancy skills which are now required.

Peter Marris (1993) refers to the fact that 'a desire to adapt to change has first to overcome an impulse to restore the past.' Within this past are three elements which make up our success or failure to manage change. They are:

- continuity
- growth
- loss.

Continuity includes patterns of expectations that remain the same, for example, moving house, changing jobs. The continuity of life is unbroken as the expectations are a means of meeting familiar needs.

Growth is in line with what would be seen as a hierarchy of needs (see p. 51). We all need shelter, food, water, clothing, comfort, company, friends, love and satisfaction. The urge to explore new kinds of satisfaction is only released when we feel confident that our more basic needs have been met. Spontaneous growth then follows from familiar patterns of expectation.

The third element, loss, can occur in many forms. Someone who loses their job might grieve not so much for their loss of job, status, money and position in society, but more for the loss of the friends they worked with. However Marris does say that when there is a crisis of discontinuity, despite the subsequent despair and sense of bereavement a new sense of purpose will eventually follow. Out of this growth occurs. If such grief is denied then loss is experienced more painfully, with loss opportunity of recovery and growth.

Scraggs *et al.* (1993) talk about the resistance to change coming from various places, for example, fear of the future, lack of information, threat to status and power, etc. It can sometimes be helpful just to list the resistances to change. Change upsets the status quo and there will always be winners and losers – it is the manager's job to try and minimise the number of losers.

Preparing for change is essential. Before implementing change it is important for a manager to consider the following questions in preparation:

- What do I need to change?
- Why?
- What's in it for me?
- Do I have a say in the change?
- Have I been kept informed of the planning stages in implementing change?
- Is it clear what change is envisaged?
- Who will benefit and who will lose out?
- Who has power and who can help with the change?

Force Field Analysis could be a useful tool here in helping to move on staff who are rigidly resisting change (see Chapter 5, p. 129).

Case study

The closing of a children's home

An example of resistance to change was the closing of a large children's home whose origins date to the 1870s. This was a very complex task which required particular sensitivity and skills, not just to deal with the organisation and staff and clients in it but also to deal with the community who viewed the home as a piece of history which they believed should not have to close and which should be supported to remain open.

From day one all staff were involved in the planning and were helped to see the need to close. Although there was a timetable for closure it was very much dictated by the plans to move children into alternative accommodation with families. Staff were supported and counselled into new jobs. It took two years to complete and when the project ended there were few if any casualties.

One of the main differences, in contrast to other experiences of closure, was connected with the external management of the project regarding the decisions made about closure. The management were prepared to put in the resources needed to close the home (closure doesn't come cheap!) They were also prepared to accept responsibility for the closure, unlike with other experiences of closure (once closure is decided upon, management often appears to disown the decision). It is like someone who dies: the surviving relative frequently suffers isolation because people do not know what to say and avoid talking to them, especially about the death. Similarly a manager closing a project has no support and has to carry the stresses and strains of the entire staff and client group on their own shoulders. In such circumstances severe problems can occur and closure becomes a very damaging experience for all.

Experiencing change is something we all do, but managing it is something only a few of us do well. Managers need to learn to be more open and less defensive and to allow their staff to play a greater part in the preparation for change. By understanding and empathising with staff managers can gain greater insight into the fear and anxiety staff are experiencing. Managers can then more successfully confront staff resistance. **Ultimately one needs to experience change to truly learn about it.**

> I hear and I forget
> I see and I remember
> I do and I understand
> (Confucius)

Reflective activity

When was the last time you experienced a major change in your life? How did you cope? Relate the theory of Organisational Change to your own experience.

Equal opportunities in management

Equal opportunities in management is about ensuring that everybody has equal access to opportunities for promotion, extra pay and better conditions, and is one of the most challenging and difficult tasks for the present-day manager. It is important to note that equal opportunities can be seen as one of the most important subjects in management because it is about one's own value system; in essence it's what you believe in. If you are managing human resources then you need a genuine belief that all people should be treated with the same degree of fairness. Of course in reality you know this is not true; human nature tells us that there will always be discrimination and prejudice. If this occurs then the manager loses out. The person being discriminated against will lose their goodwill for the organisation and conflict will soon ensue. Such conflict uses up the workforce's energy and the team's togetherness breaks down, thus diverting them from their task. Group productivity is then lost.

Most organisations have either a fully operational equal opportunities policy (EOP) or a policy of intent. An **Equal Opportunities Policy** is a statement of intent giving notice of what an organisation considers its staff should expect from it. Most EOPs are generally full of good intent like, 'We believe that all staff should be given equal access to opportunity. No staff will be discriminated against on grounds of race, gender or sexuality', etc. Yet they often fail to say how these policies will be implemented. If you believe that men are better than women, then an EOP is unlikely to force you to behave any differently. What might be different is your heightened awareness of the possibilities of subverting it. You would be more subtle in your sexist jokes about women and and would very soon learn the sophistication of hiding blatant discrimination with more indirect discrimination.

Sexism is a socially controlled phenomenon. It is to be found in the newspapers, on television and radio, in our workplaces and in every walk of life. It therefore becomes easy to accept it as part of normality and of ourselves. It takes a concerted effort to resist sexism.

Neil Thompson (1993) discusses how age and class have divided society for centuries and yet are harder to define in law than race and gender and so discrimination on grounds of age and class is more difficult to tackle. Race and gender have quite rightly been given a high profile in management and there are laws to protect people from being discriminated against on those grounds. Class values and ageism are interwoven into the fabric of society and often accepted as a part of life.

Yet it still feels difficult to accept the situation where a 28-year-old man is made redundant from the Stock Exchange and told he is too old to reapply for a similar job. This entire subject is very complex and further specialised reading is recommended. It is essential to understand the concepts before one can begin to practise in an anti-discriminatory way.

Discrimination seeps through all aspects of a manager's job and however much one tries to avoid it, it's there. The main areas where EOP has a vital role to play are in:
- Recruitment and selection
- Training
- Staff appraisal
- Supervision.

An organisation may have a policy of equal opportunities yet fails to attract the right quota of black candidates for a job because they have not advertised in the black press. The candidates who apply will be white, therefore the job will be given to a white applicant, and in defending this decision the argument 'Only white candidates applied' might be used.

You can see by examining this further that indirect discrimination takes place because you are not making the same information available to all possible candidates. Moreover if you were serious about employing a black applicant then you would probably target the black press. This is one of many examples used to demonstrate the complexity of discrimination.

If you want to be successful with people then you must begin to examine your own values and beliefs in an open way. If you discover racist or sexist beliefs it does not mean you are a bad person as this is a part of your own culture and history; what it means is that it might affect other people in a negative way. You need to be aware of this and prepared to do something about it. Equally, if a colleague is being racist or sexist then to ignore it is to collude with it and is just as discriminatory. Moreover the problem is not for minority groups to take a lead in, but for majority groups to take the lead.

Anti-discriminatory practice seeks to ensure that empowerment is to the fore, in order to ensure that social work is a progressive force for social change and amelioration rather than a repressive arm of an uncaring state bureaucracy. The challenge is a major one but the rewards for success are high, as indeed are the costs of failure. (Thompson (1993), p. 156)

Evidence opportunity

a Examine your own use of language and how this might contribute towards offending someone else.

b Discuss in groups your own beliefs and values regarding those groups which are oppressed, and where did such values come from?

c Have you experienced oppression? If so, explore the associated feelings this gave you and share them with the group.

You need to work in an honest way for this exercise to be of any real benefit.

7   The caring environment

What is covered in this chapter

- Care organisations
- Organisational culture
- Organisation structure
- Welfare State
- Reorganisation of health provision
- Differences in service provision
- National Health Service and Community Care Act 1990
- Local authority standards of care
- Registered Homes Act 1984
- Resources
- Health and safety
- Funding
- Care values
- Culture of the environment
- Empowerment
- Instruments of change
- Staffing issues

Care organisations

This chapter looks at care organisations and how they operate. To understand care organisations it is necessary to look at the history of organisations. Caring organisations have always existed for as long as there have been people who cared. However the design and purpose of care organisations was often different from those of today. It is generally recognised that the first modern caring organisations which had any real impact on modern society were not established until the mid-nineteenth century (see Tossell and Webb 1988). These were called charities from the Latin word *caritas* meaning 'regard, esteem, affection, love'.

History

The growth of the voluntary charity system was haphazard as a large range of willing groups formed to help the needy. Usually these charity groups were formed through church organisations or wealthy philanthropic (charitable) individuals. Such groups as the Salvation Army or Dr Barnardo's were examples of that time. Many vulnerable people of the time either starved or were worked to death and one of the few ways of surviving was to attend one of the many missions springing up during the 1860s and 1870s. Recipients of food and shelter had to join the Christian faith in order to get help.

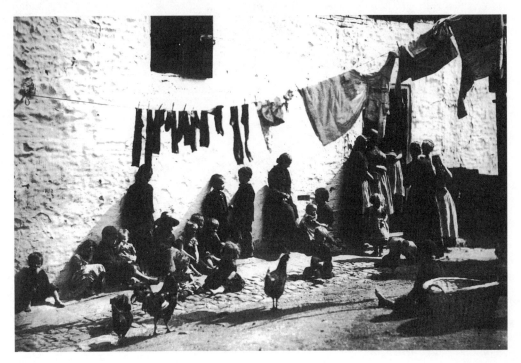

A London slum in 1889

Often food would not be given until they had first joined in with prayer.

During the nineteenth century all social services were offered by charities. There was no statutory provision. Although they still play an important role today, charities are varied and diverse, ranging from small groups of one or two people (such as counselling projects for victims of crime) to large organisations who employ thousands of people (Save the Children Fund or Age Concern).

The law relating to social services goes back to the Poor Law 1834. This law was based largely on the principle that people were poor through their own fault and to help them would only encourage 'idleness' and 'intemperance' (drunkenness). The law stated that those capable of work would no longer receive any financial assistance in their own homes. Proof of a person's destitution was that they were prepared to leave home together with members of their family and live and work in the workhouse.

Conditions were deliberately made harsh and families were split up as the rules were made uncompromising. Those administrators of the time failed to understand that poverty and illness were directly linked to living conditions. Such beliefs were perpetuated through the legislation of that time. The Beveridge Report of 1942 led to the creation of the Welfare State and the beginning of the voluntary sector's (charities') relationship with state provision. Before 1942 it was the voluntary movement which acted as society's conscience. War-time conditions forced the British government into legislating and providing everyone with the same social benefits on a free basis.

In 1968 an important report (the Seebohm Report) led to major changes in the structure

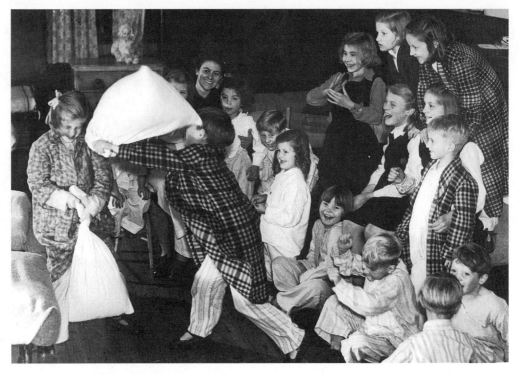

Scene from a Dr. Barnardo's home in 1950: the Second World War brought changes in attitudes to social care

of social services. It was as a result of this that a law was passed in 1970 (Social Services Act 1970) establishing the social services as they exist today headed by a Director who is responsible for local authority services. Previously social services were divided into departments; consequently you might have a children's social worker and welfare social worker attending the same house: one interested in the child, the other in the parents, yet not liaising with each other. This legislation brought them all together.

Social services have undergone another change which has significantly developed their relationship with the private and voluntary sectors; this change is known as Community Care. Moving people out of institutions and into the community whether they live independently or with their families or friends, is what Community Care is all about. It is no new concept and has been about since the Mental Deficiency Act 1913 when it was suggested that long-stay mentally ill people might be better off living with someone else if they were not a risk to society. Much debate followed through the years. The Barclay Report 1980 (a government working party) made some recommendations about people in need being provided with care in the community. Following this another report (Griffiths Report 1988) made firm proposals to restructure how need should be assessed, care delivered and financed and resources gained. The NHS and Community Care Act 1990 took up many of Griffiths' recommendations and local authorities were forced into rebuilding their infrastructure to take account of these changes (redeveloping how they worked).

(For a brief outline of these changes please see the *A-B-C of Community Care* by Harry Tunnicliffe *et al.*, 1993)

How many caring voluntary organisations or groups do you know of? Do they supplement, add to, or complement (do the same things) what the local authority social services offer?

Private caring organisations have always been around, often as nursing or convalescent homes. The National Health Service and Community Care Act 1990 made it compulsory for local authorities to buy private residential home care with up to 62 per cent of their total budget. There has been a major shift in government policy towards opting out of statutory sector provision and moving into the private sector as it opens up a free market. A free market allows a buyer of services to purchase from wherever they wish, which in reality means opting for the cheapest that can still maintain quality and standards. The notion of competition was believed to be the major force behind achieving quality at a reasonable price. This has been a lasting principle from the 1980s. One of the main criticisms of the previous system of purchasing was that authorities used their own services. A local authority would employ many people, which often caused duplication of work and ultimately public funding was wasted.

Local authorities began to contract private care organisations to run large sections of the social services, for example, domiciliary services (meals on wheels, home care, etc.) or residential homes for the elderly. Large companies were beginning to invest in this area as they saw it as a way of making money and expanding the market. More importantly for the government private care created competition, which meant that some of the smaller homes would have to increase standards if they wished to compete. The government's hope was that while the private companies were making money they would also be contracted to certain specifications and deliver a quality service to ensure standards would be maintained and bettered. To help assess this, the government adopted a new concept which you will begin to hear a great deal about; it is known as **quality indicators**. Quality indicators are used to measure whether or not an organisation has achieved targets (a sort of yardstick).

As the purchaser of the service the local authority has the power to revoke (close) the contract if the supplier does not come up to scratch. The local authority can tender for a new contract with a different organisation. The theory of this is that it will benefit the customer/client/patient.

Ask the opinions of a range of staff who work in different organisations which have been affected by the NHS and Community Care reforms and reflect on their views as to whether in practice the public are now better off since the implementation of Community Care.

Changes gradually brought about a shift in the main providers of social services from the voluntary groups up to the 1940s to the statutory services between 1948 and 1979. Since the latest community care legislation there has been yet another move resulting in some services being supplied by only the private sector (e.g. meals on wheels, residential care, etc.).

Evidence opportunity

One of the aims of the Community Care reforms is 'Value for Money'; examine what the different issues are for statutory local authorities, voluntary organisations and private organisations which offer social care. Try to establish whether the difference in these issues affects the notion of 'Value for Money'.

This chapter now examines how the three different types of caring organisations, voluntary, private and statutory operate.

Voluntary organisations

As already mentioned the main motivation and goals of voluntary organisations are about achieving what might be described as a better way of life for vulnerable people. Such an organisation has no legal powers or duties to provide services but when providing services it must operate within the law. For example, if an organisation is running a children's home, the way it is run must comply with the Children Act 1989 and subsequent guidance (HMSO Vol. 4). This makes the way it operates subject to legal requirements. There are also other laws which require financial operations to be scrutinised (or reviewed) in public. For example, the Charity Commission which oversees voluntary organisations is a government body which must establish whether or not such an organisation is fit to continue running. All such organisations rely on voluntarily donated income and raising money through charitable events. The organisation must be made accountable for the money raised. All voluntary groups must publish their accounts annually. Charities must register and will be given a charity number which gives them legal status entitling them to raise funds through charitable events. The benefits of charitable status include exemption from VAT in some areas and tax free profits, all of which must go back into the organisation.

Voluntary organisations are normally run by a board of governors, committee, trustees or council. These are all democratically elected posts. However, organisations such as Barnardo's view themselves as being non-political and therefore believe that all members are essentially committed to the work of the organisation. The organisation appoints a director to run the operation who has to report back to the council. This process is becoming more complicated as organisations struggle to survive in a recession and are forced to undertake more commercially motivated operations, such as the charity shops which raise a useful amount of income.

These shops are self financing and are run like businesses. They have very little in the way of outgoings as all the staff are volunteers. The premises are normally rented on low cost short-term leases, or in some cases the building is owned by the organisation, such investment increasing their capital for a future date.

Evidence opportunity

How many charity shops are there in your area? This may give you an indication as to what extent they are seen as money raisers.

A voluntary organisation runs in a similar way to a private company. Some care workers find the mix of commercial profitability and meeting the needs of vulnerable people unpalatable to the social care task. For example, investing in the corporate image of a large organisation takes a lot of money. This is essential in order to put across their message to the general public so that people will want to donate money to their caring charity. On the other hand workers in the organisation may see this as a waste of the organisation's money and may think that the £200,000 invested on advertising could have been better spent on buying, say, a new residential home for six disabled young people.

This is only one of many current moral dilemmas such organisations struggle with daily.

Evidence opportunity

Discuss this with your colleagues and identify the points for and against commercial and voluntary links. Do you see any moral or ethical issues here?

Reflective activity

Reflect on where you stand in the debate on commercial approaches to social care.

Because a voluntary organisation has no politically elected group nor private shareholders with vested interests, theoretically this should leave it free to take risks and be more creative. Many of the specialist services are voluntary because they have been able to do the pioneering work and build up their expertise. Such expertise is now offered to statutory and private agencies as a way of generating income, thus allowing the voluntary agencies to continue at a time when cutbacks in grants are forcing many voluntary organisations to close.

For example, Barnardo's was one of the first to accept HIV infected children into residential care whilst many other places either did not have a policy or for other reasons were unable to help. They were able to take a risk in what was at the time (1989) a controversial area. In another example the Children's Society was the first to take the risk of providing a safe house for runaway children (1988). At the time any organisation harbouring runaway children would be acting illegally and therefore breaking the law (this did not apply to Scotland where it was legal).

Their risk and campaigning paid off because just before the implementation of the Children Act 1989 amendments were made to include safe houses under this law with new regulations. There are many other examples where voluntary groups and organisations are able to specialise and take risks, thus paving the way for others to follow just as they did in the nineteenth century.

Although voluntary groups and organisations have a major role to play in providing services they are seen as being similar to local authorities in their accountability. For example, under quality control requirements all residential homes must, by law, be inspected; this was made to safeguard client rights and ensure the homes were properly run in the context of value for money and a quality service. So certain legislation regarding the control and running of residential homes covers all homes whatever sector they fall into.

Private organisations

These are set up purely to make a profit. They are normally run on the basis of one person being in charge who has much more power than say a director of a local authority or voluntary organisation – because they own the company or are a major shareholder or are accountable to shareholders who normally have little interest in the running of the project (as their interest is purely in the amount of profit they will make). For example, a shareholder might not get involved unless the project was not making the profits they expected. A manager would normally only be judged on their ability to sustain profit growth rather than to deliver a quality service.

In the 1990s the private sector is an area that is expanding due to the present government's initiative on free market economics. In a caring context profit does not always sit nicely with the task of caring. However, there are many examples of good quality nursing homes which are better run by private establishments. One of the reasons for this is that they often have the financial capital to invest in a large way. In an average authority they might have up to fifteen residential homes and an average occupancy of 75 per cent. This means they are losing a potential 25 per cent on empty beds. This may be for many reasons, such as:

- the home is in the wrong area;
- the demand for such provision is lower than the rate at which beds become available;
- under the new law, people can choose where they want to live and they can exercise that right by opting to live outside the borough.

Because of these factors many local authorities contract out the running of all their residential services to a private organisation. By this means, they do not have to take on the financial liabilities of running a home (i.e. keeping open a home which is not financially viable). The risk is transferred to the new organisation. Many small private homes are struggling since they are not able to provide care at the cost local authorities require in their specifications, without going out of business.

The answer is simple: large companies, often with no care experience, buy up all the small homes and run them under a large corporation. Because of their size they can afford to run homes more economically and therefore are more likely to win local authority contracts and maintain a higher bed occupancy level. Because they are cheaper they will be used more often and also are not restricted to a particular geographical area and can therefore advertise nationally.

There are many reported negative sides to this. Once a company creates a monopoly of care over other suppliers they are in a powerful position to drop standards by cutting back on staff or paying lower wages to increase their profit margins. However, there could be benefits, in that staff are paid some of the profits the company makes, or are remunerated through what is becoming an increasing practice – profit related pay. Staff have to achieve certain targets (normally set to standards) to qualify for a bonus, or (in some cases) to qualify for their standard rate of pay. Either way all these systems of rewarding staff for greater effort are open to abuse. It comes down to the major shareholder or owner deciding how the operation will run and in cases of conflict there is very little an individual can do unless the employer has broken the law, or there is an agreement between the employer and one of the trade unions.

You may have experienced this change in financial ownership in many areas of what used to be the public services. For example, the way schools now take over their own budget and run their own affairs. Many of the boards of governors have co-opted onto

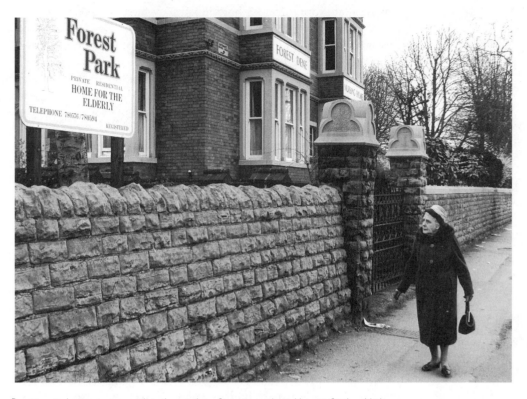

Recent years have seen a growth in the number of private residential homes for the elderly

the school's governing body people with commercial backgrounds such as accountants or lawyers rather than educators. Another good example is in the National Health Service where a hospital can opt out and take trust status. Again the area health authorities who would normally be responsible for hospitals have changed as hospitals become self-managing. Business people with a commercial background are used to manage the trusts rather than the medical consultants as management becomes increasingly about managing money rather than care.

Reflective activity

Can you think of any other public service you use whose financial status has changed now that they have their own budget and can buy services from anywhere they want?

Statutory organisations

Statutory organisations must provide certain services because the law directs them to do so. The structure, design and activities these organisations are engaged in are required by law.

To understand this you need to know something about local government. Local representatives of an area are elected to the council where they serve four years in office. They are responsible through various committees for overseeing and financing various public services such as social services, transport, housing, etc.

The local authority decides how much they have to spend which often dictates what services will be provided or what will be cut. The spending levels are complex as they rely on the amount of grant given to them by central government; the government decides this grant by taking into account whether there is an overspend or not, as well as the amount of council tax collected. All these considerations influence the final amount a council has to spend. Then it is up to each individual council committee to negotiate money for their special interest. Social services will be given a budget and it is up to the director and officers to prioritise their expenditure.

This entire area is complex but it is important to mention some of the dilemmas being faced in relation to funding.

- Stability versus Flexibility – purchasers want flexibility in where and when they buy services so that they can be more user and needs led, but providers want some guarantees of financial stability to enable them to stay in business.
- Competition versus Cooperation – purchasers want to force prices down, especially in residential care, whilst providers are less happy with such market tactics. Small homes are more likely to be forced out of business because they will not be able to lower their prices and compete.
- Preferred Providers versus Open Purchasers – should purchasers rely on known reliable providers or go to the open market?
- Political Control versus Needs Led Services – is it the duty of purchasers to follow political directives as to what services should be bought or should decisions be solely user driven?

There are of course many more dilemmas having to be faced daily by purchasers and providers of care but these limited examples will perhaps highlight the complexity of these changes.

Other new legislation has also had an impact on how local authorities have changed. For example, the Children Act 1989 and the Criminal Justice Act 1991 require local authorities to undertake certain activities with young people which will inevitably involve cost. Local authorities have little choice.

Below are two examples which demonstrate the problem.

Before the Children Act 1989 and the Criminal Justice Act 1991 were implemented the government made an amount of money available to all local authorities to help prepare for their new responsibilities. There were hidden costs. Under the Children Act 1989 a duty was imposed on local authorities to provide a fully accessible representation and complaints procedure. As a result many young people used these complaints procedures to complain. Local authorities planned for the financial costs of employing a complaints officer, adjudicating officer and investigating officer, essential to fulfil their service, but did not plan for the independent person.

Each complaint must by law be overseen by an independent person. Their time costs money which local authorities are forced to find by taking from another budget. A hidden cost.

Under the new Criminal Justice Act 1991 a young person under sixteen years of age is the responsibility of their parents and a court may fine the parents for their child's delinquent behaviour. Some local authorities who are acting as parents through having children in care have been taken to court and fined many hundreds of pounds because the child is out of control.

Consequently local authorities have little power or control in how they spend their money. To a certain extent local authorities are viewed by the electorate as having to

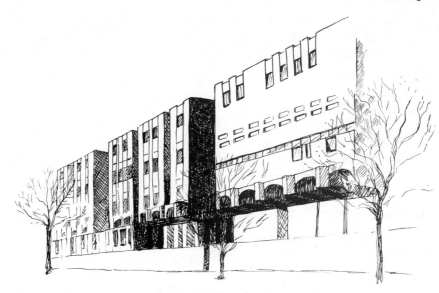

Modern social services offices

honour election pledges and meet locally identified needs, but more importantly, they have to carry out central government directives and duties enforced by legal requirements. Because in a recession money becomes harder to find, cutbacks become more inevitable. Many local authorities have been forced into providing the bare minimum required under the law. Much health and social care legislation gives a power to provide a service, but in reality the service becomes the most likely area to cut back. Much of the preventative work which was normally done under legislative powers is being cut by local authorities and taken up by voluntary groups.

For example, in very cold weather social workers used to visit elderly people to ensure they were warm and were being fed; now it's left to neighbours or voluntary groups such as Age Concern to mobilise a group of volunteers to visit.

Statutory organisations carry out tasks and functions as required by law and in times of cutbacks will only do the minimum required by such law. This is why so often they are unable to take financial risks or be creative like the private and voluntary organisations since they have neither the means nor resources to do so.

Much of the statutory work undertaken by many different authorities is being opened up for debate in order to find ways to save money. Privatisation is one option. For example, the government has explored ways in which prisons can be privately run.

Reflective activity

Is there anything wrong in saving taxpayers' money to provide a cheaper service? In providing a service with a limited budget what factors should not be compromised?

Organisational culture

According to Charles Handy (1985) all organisations have a culture known as an 'organisation culture'. Understanding this culture is essential to understanding how organisations work. This culture is different to the type of culture referred to when talking about a particular residential home or group of people. Here we mean organisations. According to Charles Handy, organisations have either one culture or a combination of cultures.

Power culture

The power culture (also known as Zeus) has a web-like structure. The Spider in the middle dominates and controls everything around. Everyone in the web is controlled by this mighty powerful leader who rules by whim and impulse. The managing director of a large company who assumes this culture would act like a tyrant (oppressive ruler).

Role culture

The role culture (also known as Apollo) has a structure like a Greek temple. Managers rule by logic and reason. Their strengths are in having systems for everything and a rule book which prescribes all you need to know. People in this culture are known as a role and not a person (the Civil Service is a good example, as you may be known for your grade and not your name).

Task culture

The task culture has a structure like a net with some of the strands thicker than others. Power and influence lie where the strands join in the net, perhaps at the knot. The emphasis is on getting the job done. Such a culture is often associated with experts or people who come in to do a job on a short-term basis, such as management consultants.

Person culture

The person culture (also known as Dionysus) is structured like a cluster. The cluster concept is based on the image of a cluster of stars: people in an organisation who have expert knowledge and therefore power. Barristers or consultant physicians might be professional groups who operate in this way – together they form powerful groups.

As one might expect there is a lot more to this, which can be read in Handy's book, *Understanding Organisations* (1985). Handy also gives a very useful exercise on organisational culture that the reader can easily complete. The exercise explicitly helps to identify one's preferred culture, and if you are working in an agency the culture the organisation adopts (1985 pp. 214–221).

Understanding the organisation you study in or work for can be vital to understanding how to effect change. All organisations have a preferred culture, and if as an individual you are attempting to change something in a particular organisation, you will have severe problems if you go against that culture. Understanding management can help you avoid many of the disastrous pitfalls.

Evidence opportunity

Think about the organisation you either work or study in. Is there a dominant culture you can identify? Discuss this with your friends, tutors and colleagues at college.

A diagrammatic view of organisation structure

The following is a selection of diagrams to show how some organisations are structured in their hierarchy and therefore power. Because of the increasing amount of restructuring in local authorities it is difficult to offer universal examples as structures keep changing. The following diagrams will give an indication of structure.

A private organisation structure

Because most private care organisations are small they normally only represent the owner and workers. The following example is of a large company.

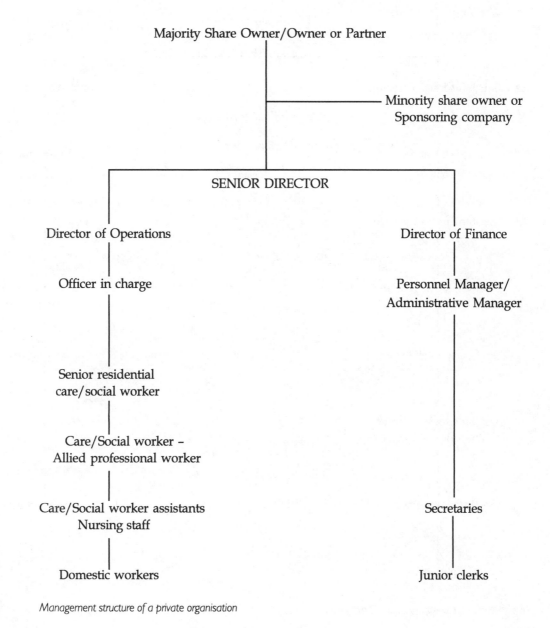

Management structure of a private organisation

A voluntary organisation structure

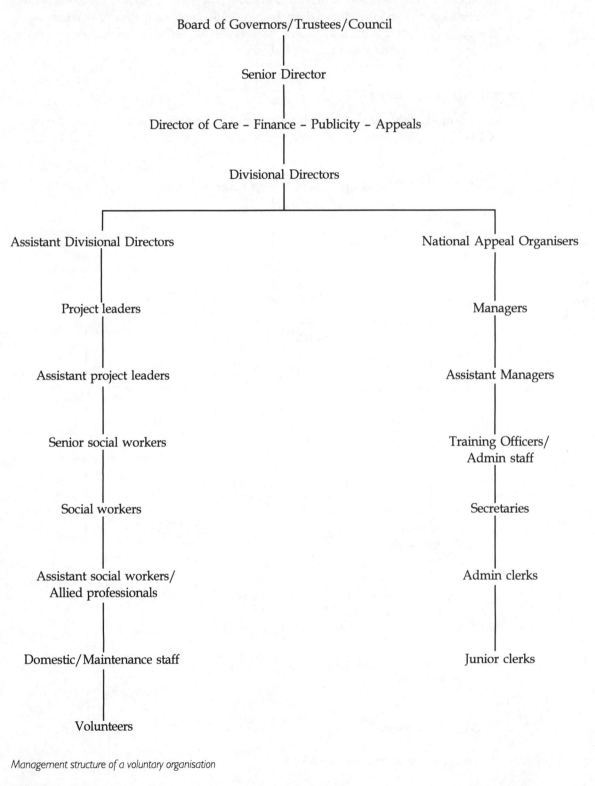

Management structure of a voluntary organisation

A statutory organisation structure

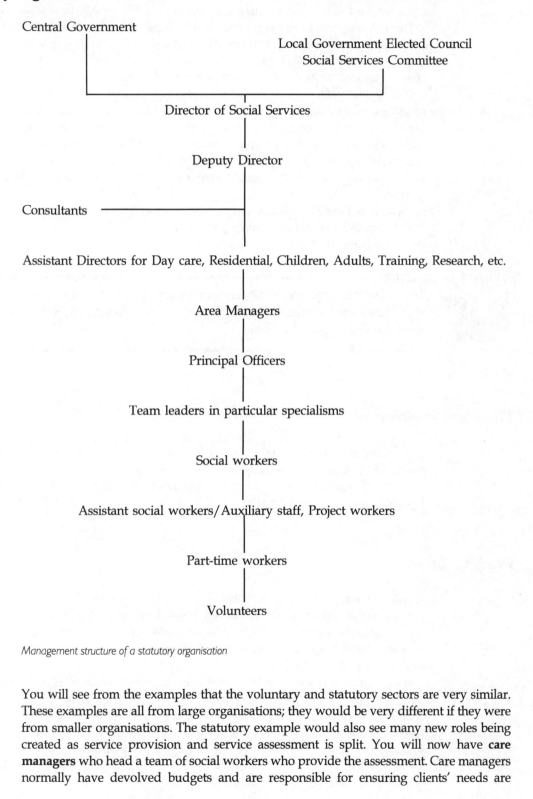

Central Government

Local Government Elected Council
Social Services Committee

Director of Social Services

Deputy Director

Consultants

Assistant Directors for Day care, Residential, Children, Adults, Training, Research, etc.

Area Managers

Principal Officers

Team leaders in particular specialisms

Social workers

Assistant social workers/Auxiliary staff, Project workers

Part-time workers

Volunteers

Management structure of a statutory organisation

You will see from the examples that the voluntary and statutory sectors are very similar. These examples are all from large organisations; they would be very different if they were from smaller organisations. The statutory example would also see many new roles being created as service provision and service assessment is split. You will now have **care managers** who head a team of social workers who provide the assessment. Care managers normally have devolved budgets and are responsible for ensuring clients' needs are identified. Care managers are also responsible for working out a package of care which offers the best value (within quality maintained levels and the new legal framework.)

There would also be someone responsible at principal officer level for managing purchasing services. They would ensure they make all the right contacts with provider agencies to strike the best deal (gain the best cost for a service). You may also see examples of decentralised reorganisation where field work offices move out of the large council premises into small ones in the community. For example, in London there are several councils (Tower Hamlets, Islington) who use what are called 'One Stop Shops' where a person can call for information or advice on housing, finance or social care problems all under one roof, instead of having to be referred to different offices all over the borough. Within this system it is normally a general manager who has overall control of the operations and reports to a chief executive who may or may not have a social work background.

For a more detailed look at social care organisations and community services please see *Introduction to Social and Community Services* (1992) by W.E. Baugh and *Social Welfare Alive* (1993) by Stephen Moore.

Evidence opportunity

Try to find out what system of statutory structure operates in your area. Look at your local social services and examine how they are structured. Reflect on whether what you find is a good system.

The care environment

This part of the chapter looks at the caring environment noting the resources available to create and maintain care settings in the statutory, voluntary, public and private sectors. Policies and legislation which affect care organisations will be explored and opportunities to collect evidence will be given.

Welfare State

It will be useful to review briefly the creation of the Welfare State when considering the provision of health and care. The starting point is the Beveridge Report of 1942 which was instrumental in creating the Welfare State in 1948 to rid the country of 'the five giants of want, disease, ignorance, squalor and idleness' for every citizen of the UK from the cradle to the grave.

As a result a series of legislation was enacted: the National Health Service Bill in 1946 which became law in 1948, the Housing Act 1946 and the Education Act 1944. In 1974 Health and Social Services became two separate provisions. A range of supplementary legislation has led to the National Health Service and Community Care Act in 1990. This radically changes the provision of care through a gradual move away from state responsibility for the provision of health and personal social service care to individual responsibility with state support if necessary.

Reorganisation of health provision

During her term in office, Margaret Thatcher's Conservative government produced a White Paper 'Working for Patients: the National Health Service Caring for the 1990s'. The White Paper sought to provide an expanded service to meet the needs of a growing population who were enjoying better health and living longer than in the 1940s when the Welfare State was conceived. The aim was to provide a more efficient and effective service which put patients first.

As a result of the White Paper, Health Service provision is undergoing a complete organisational change with the emphasis placed on budget controls for all areas. For example, within a large hospital all departments have a budget which must be adhered to in order to provide that service. If the manager underestimates or does not allow for error, then that department may have to close in part or in whole until the next financial year. It should be remembered that hospitals are themselves both purchasers and providers of services.

The country is divided into sixteen Regional Health Authorities who provide operational plans for their area and are responsible to the Secretary of State at the Department of Health. Each region is subdivided into District Health Authorities whose role is to assess the need of the residents in the district and to buy in the services they require either from hospitals in their own district or from another district if the specialist provision is unavailable locally. The keywords are cost effective health care. The positive side for the patient is that they have a right to make a case to use the service most suitable for their needs.

Hospitals and community units are providers of services which the District Health Authority may use, or not use, depending on the patient's need and the cost involved compared with alternative providers. The whole philosophy is that money should follow patients and not the other way round.

Hospital trusts

Some larger hospitals have elected to apply for trust status. This means that a given hospital may apply to the Department of Health for hospital trust status. The hospital must provide a viable business plan to demonstrate that it is capable of maintaining its level of service at or above minimum standards for service provision within its budget. If trust status is granted then the trust is responsible directly to the Department of Health, thus bypassing the Regional Health Authorities.

Family health service authority

A new Family Health Service Authority purchases the services of dentists, opticians, pharmacists and general practitioners within its area. Some general practitioners have opted to become fund holders and take their funds directly from the Regional Health Authority rather than the Family Health Service Authority. Such fund holders buy in the services of staff, e.g. district nurses, for their patients as and when necessary.

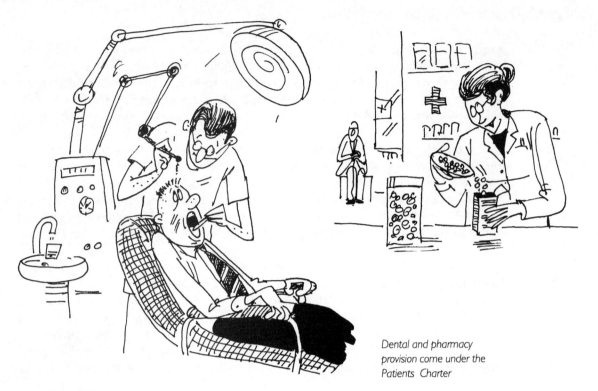

Dental and pharmacy
provision come under the
Patients Charter

Patients Charter

A Patients Charter was produced by the Conservative government setting out nine National Charter standards which staff, patients and relatives/friends should become familiar with. April 1992 saw the introduction of three new rights concerning data on the efficiency and quality of local health services, complaints procedures and waiting time for treatment. These three new rights at local level place a responsibility on service providers to publish relevant data; for example, in an Accident and Emergency unit there should be details of waiting times for treatment after assessment. The District Health Authority has to publish an annual report showing achievements against the local standards set.

Evidence opportunity

Visit your local hospital and/or health centre to find out the targets set for each. Note the evidence displayed of achievements to date. Have local targets been met? If not see if you are able to find out what the constraints were. Discuss your findings in a group.

On the social care side, it is estimated that approximately 14 per cent of the UK population in the 1990s will be receiving care in their own home from informal carers, i.e. from family, neighbours and friends. Others will need support in residential settings whether for health reasons involving the National Health Service, or for care and protection as in childcare services, or due to age or disability.

Residential care and day care services are provided by three different types of care organisations described earlier in the chapter:

- **Statutory**: the structure of the different departments that come under this heading are laid down by law, e.g. Social Services providing care for elders or places of safety for children.
- **Private**: here a need has been identified, e.g. residential care for elders, and a business has been set up to meet that demand. Private homes aim to provide care but need to make a profit whilst caring for a specific group. Care is provided which has to comply with the minimum standards laid down by the National Health Service and Community Care Act 1990. The cost has to be realistic and set at a rate that the market in the area can bear.
- **Voluntary**: this sector may be organised on a local or national level. An individual or group of individuals have identified a need which is currently not being fully met by the statutory services. Volunteers work to raise funds to provide a service which complements the work of the statutory services, e.g. a local support group for parents of children with particular disabilities may set up a playgroup and advice centre. Barnardos is a national charity providing care for children. Voluntary groups register with the Charities Commission.

All health and care organisations are currently under financial pressure to be more cost effective. Staff may feel that the quality of service they are able to provide is being adversely affected by budget restrictions. This may well lead to a feeling of powerlessness and inadequacy, 'I know what I would like to do but the resources are just not available!'

Evidence opportunity

Arrange an interview with a service provider. Find out what the main issues are without going into details concerning actual finance which may well be a sensitive issue. Look at what the provider wishes to do and what they are able to do. Analyse your findings by discussion in the group. Do remember the issues regarding confidentiality during this exercise.

One of the most important issues is to ensure that any changes envisaged are communicated clearly to all staff. Team meetings where staff are encouraged to discuss their concerns in a constructive manner may help to ensure that staff feel they are able to understand and contribute to the running of the unit.

Differences in service provision

It must be remembered that different organisations make different demands on staff groups. A social care worker in the statutory sector may find that their role has many similarities to that performed by a care worker in the private sector. In the private sector there may be additional roles regarding cooking and cleaning in some residential settings. Cooking and cleaning are not part of the work of a social worker in the statutory sector.

Voluntary organisations often have many volunteers rather than paid care staff. This makes different demands on the staff group in terms of management and organisation. Managers must ensure that the service is coordinated and maintains the required standard of care expected by the clients.

Statutory services obtain their funds from a central budget held by the local authority in the case of social services establishments or by hospital trustees in the Health Service. Voluntary organisations will have a board of trustees who control fund raising and apply for any grants possible from central government or local authorities or other fund raising events such as Telethon.

Very large organisations, whether they are private, statutory or voluntary, have even more complex problems in the management and organisation of several groups of staff and clients. Staff may find that they are moved from one unit to another. Staff have to adapt to a new group and learn the norms and values including the culture of the group. This will be necessary in order to be accepted and to enable cooperative work to get the job done.

Change can be stressful and result in an individual feeling isolated, undervalued and demotivated. Strategies are needed to assist the individual to cope with the situation. Teamwork is one of two models of working in groups. A team, as we have seen, is a group of people working in close proximity to each other, for example the staff in a small family group home.

Evidence opportunity

What are the factors essential to create a caring environment? You might write down your thoughts in a list and compare notes with a colleague on the programme. You may wish to talk to staff in a variety of health and care settings. You may also wish to talk to service users and gain an insight into their point of view.

What you will probably find is a wide range of answers. These could be used to draw out the essential factors considered necessary to provide a caring environment.

The National Health Service and Community Care Act 1990

The National Health Service and Community Care Act 1990 transferred the responsibility for the funding of new customers for residential and nursing homes from the Department of Social Security to local authorities. Each local authority had to prepare a specification of Standards for Care. You may wish to view a copy of the standards produced by your own local authority.

Local authority standards of care

In general the Standards for Care prepared by local authorities cover the principles and practices essential to ensuring that an individual's right to choice, citizenship, independence, personal fulfilment, dignity, privacy and equality of opportunity is maintained.

Home Life: a code of practice for residential care and *Homes are for Living in* are two documents used as the criteria for ensuring quality of care is provided. You might spend time familiarising yourself with these two important documents.

Registered Homes Act 1984

All residential settings must comply with the Registered Homes Act 1984, i.e. the minimum standard outlined by this Act must be achieved in order to be registered and to remain registered with a local authority. This means that any provider of residential care in a particular local authority whether they are private, voluntary, local authority or homes under Royal Charter, e.g. Royal National Institute for the Deaf (RNID), must be registered with their local authority. A list of all registered homes is available for anyone to see in each local authority.

Inspectorate

By law local authority Registration Officers must inspect registered homes not less than once every twelve months, although it is recommended that more frequent visits would be advantageous. A newly registered home should be visited within three months of the original registration, as should any home where a new manager has been appointed.

The purpose of inspection is to ensure that the quality of care provided meets minimum standards as outlined in *Home Life: a code of practice for residential care*, and to review the management of the establishment. A written report is sent to the home following each inspection highlighting any issue that had arisen and making recommendations for improvement if necessary.

Client rights/equal opportunities

A checklist is used as a guide for the inspection covering such aspects as number and movements of residents, record keeping, health and social care, community links, staffing in terms of the number and appropriateness of qualifications, catering facilities, general condition of the premises and the management of the home. Care is taken to ensure that the rights of the residents are being maintained, particularly with regard to needs in terms of religion, culture or ethnicity. Registration Officers must have free and confidential discussions with any resident who may wish to discuss the home on the visit.

Reflective activity ————————————————————————————————

Think of a residential setting that you are familiar with. Look at the client group in terms of gender and ethnicity, and compare that with the gender and ethnicity of the staff group. Are there for example any black or Asian staff to support any black or Asian clients?

Evidence opportunity ————————————————————————————————

Discuss in a group session your findings and try to explain the possible impact on a client's self-concept, on finding that they are in a minority in a particular setting. What implications do minority or isolated residents have for the staff group?

This is not an ideal world and it may be that you have not had reason to address this issue before. It is an important issue and one that will become a point of concern for many residential settings in Britain in the future. It could be that you find that there is a gender or ethnic imbalance and it is important that you are aware of the problems of discrimination, and the effect on the individual particularly in terms of self-esteem.

Evidence opportunity

Arrange a visit to a residential home. Try and find out how staff work to meet individual need in terms of ethnicity, religion and culture.

- Is it possible to provide for someone for whom English is a second language?
- Are codes of dress, dietary needs or eating practices recognised and respected?
- Is there a directory giving information regarding religious practices and including names and addresses of religious leaders or cultural groups?
- Are positive images of gender and ethnicity to be found in books, videos, music, pictures and papers supplied in the establishment?

You may wish to discuss your findings in a group and look at possible implications of your findings for staff and residents.

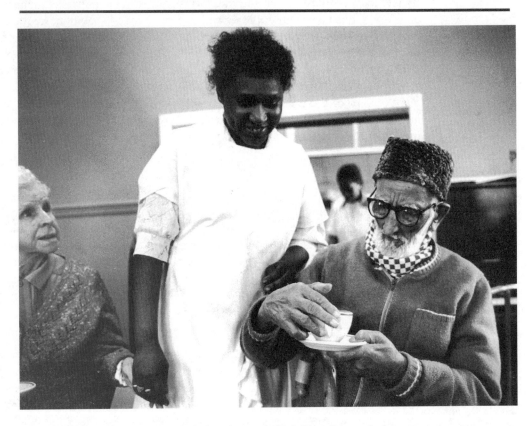

Residential homes will have to meet individual needs in terms of ethnicity, religion and culture

You may find it helpful to look again at these issue which are addressed in both mandatory Unit 1, Access Equal Opportunity and Client Rights, and mandatory Unit 4, Psychological and Social Aspects of Health and Social Care.

Resources

What are the resources necessary to provide a service for a residential home for elders? The starting point is the building as this will determine the number of residents it is possible to accommodate. Buildings come under the Buildings Regulations 1976 (SI 1976 No. 176).

The local authority provides guidelines on the space necessary for each person; for example, the minimum space for a single bedroom should be 10 square metres and one London borough advocates allocating 15.5 square metres for a double room. The said borough also recommends that every room should have its own washbasin with running hot and cold water and that no more than one fifth of residents should be accommodated in double rooms.

It is more difficult to generalise about the ratio of staff to residents as it depends on the need of the client group. An example is the general formula (London guidelines) which recommends a minimum of thirteen day-care hours per resident per week. There must be at least two members of staff on duty at a time during the day excluding the officer on shift. At night there must be a minimum of two staff awake and one sleeping in officer.

This provides only a guide as consideration must be given to the needs of the client group, i.e. residents requiring more physical help will require more staff on duty than those who are more physically active and independent. A registered first aider should be working on each shift.

Reflective activity

Think about the staffing of care settings. Take note of the earlier exercise to determine the qualities needed by a carer as perceived by a client. How might the above formula work? What limitations can you see?

Consideration must be give to the needs of individuals who wish to live at an establishment. A resident's physical needs may require that handrails be provided along corridors, in the toilet and in the bathroom. This may meet the needs of those who have difficulty in walking or maintaining their balance, for example. Lifts and ramps may be necessary; telephones, staff call bells, light switches and door handles may need to be adapted for people in wheelchairs or who have poor grip.

Architects may need to liaise with occupational therapists. Occupational therapists have expert knowledge of the needs of people with disabilities but it is important to note that special adaptations may have to be provided for a particular individual. Occupational therapists will always advise on what equipment may be bought or borrowed from social services departments or hospitals, in order to meet a particular need.

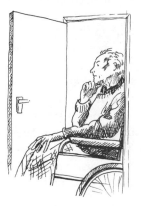

Buildings must give access to people in wheelchairs

The number of toilets and baths/showers for the number of residents is laid down in the Local Authority Specification Standards for Residential Care. At least one bathroom for every ten residents is needed. Where possible this should include a toilet and wash-basin covering an area of 9.4 square metres.

Care must be taken to ensure that access for wheelchairs is available in at least one bathroom and that residents can preserve their dignity by not having to walk through communal areas to reach the toilet. A ratio of one toilet of 2.8 square metres minimum space for every four residents is recommended. A ready supply of toilet tissue and a hand basin with running hot and cold water must be provided in every toilet as must hand drying facilities. A separate toilet must be provided for staff and all toilets must be well ventilated.

Safety locks on toilets and bathrooms should be provided so that in an emergency they may be opened quickly. A bell to call staff must be located within easy access of the toilet and in the bathroom as well as in bedrooms and communal rooms.

If commodes are to be used then each commode must be for the exclusive use of one resident and if that person shares a room there must be curtains/screen to provide privacy.

Communal rooms need to be carefully planned to ensure that there is adequate space and that there is consideration of possible safety hazards, for example, occasional tables are preferable to low coffee tables. The height and types of easy chairs and the provision of smoking and non-smoking lounges will be important to meet individual need. For instance, a person with mobility problems may need a higher chair which will not slide back when rising or sitting down.

Care needs to be taken to provide an area for quiet relaxation as well as an area for activities, television and listening to music.

Dining areas should be laid out so that there are no more than four residents to a table (1.39 square metres per person is recommended). It is important to ensure that the tables and chairs are designed in such a way that all residents may use them with ease. The layout of the dining room has to take into consideration the mobility of the residents.

Carpets, curtains and wall decorations including pictures should provide a 'homely' environment. Coffee and tea making facilities should be available at all times in a designated space that has been designed to meet health and safety requirements.

Kitchens must comply with the regulations laid down by the local Environmental Health Officer taking into consideration

- the Health and Safety Acts of 1974 and 1981
- the Food Hygiene (General) Regulations 1970
- the Food Safety Act 1990
- the Food Premises (Registration) Regulations 1991.

Care must be taken to meet the dietary needs of all residents. Special consideration must be given to specific requirements regarding the preparation and cooking of food in observance of particular religions; for example, Hindus require different sinks, bowls and knives for the preparation and cooking of vegetarian food from those used for the preparation of meat.

Heating of the building must maintain the temperature at 21 C during the day and 18 C during the night. There should be no portable heaters for health and safety reasons but individual rooms should have a thermostat on radiators to allow the individual to vary the temperature in their particular bedroom. The maximum surface temperature must not exceed 43 C or radiator guards must be fitted to prevent accidental burns.

Lifts are to be provided if the building is more than one storey high and stair wells must be well lit; there should be wide stairs (76.2 cm usable tread) with handrails on both sides.

Health and safety

The residential setting must have a current fire certificate. Regular fire drills must be held to ensure that all staff know the procedure for dealing with fire and the procedure for evacuating the building. Fire equipment must be regularly checked and a record kept of all fire drills. Appliances must be inspected and a certificate of sufficiency of gas installations within the building obtained from the supplier.

Fire alarms should be designed to meet individual need; for example, flashing lights should be installed for those who are hearing impaired in addition to bells and emergency lighting. Stairs and corridors must be kept free of obstruction and fire doors and escapes checked regularly.

The siting of the residential setting in the local area should be given consideration to ensure ease of access for visitors and to encourage the residents to be actively involved in the local community if they so wish. Parking for visitors and staff, and grounds for residents to use in fine weather should also be carefully planned. Planners will also have to decide whether bedrooms are for single occupants or are shared facilities. A major factor here will be the philosophy of the establishment. The question may be whether the residential establishment is to be developed as small units, or as a large unit with some public sitting areas and communal dining facilities.

So far new residential settings have been considered but many establishments have to adapt existing buildings to meet changing need and philosophy of care. In the sixties and seventies most residential establishments were large, with bedrooms shared by two people. People may or may not have known each other before they took up residence. Hospitals had long wards of perhaps thirty beds called Nightingale wards.

Reflective activity

How do you think an elder may feel when discovering that her new home means sharing a bedroom with someone she does not know? What effect might this have on her self-esteem?

Funding

Funding of residential places can be quite complex. For example, an older woman will have been assessed by a social worker to determine her physical, emotional, psychological and financial needs when together they explored possible options for the future.

Once the decision to enter a residential setting is made the woman can decide where she would like to go. The local authority has a register of all residential settings and will also have an 'approved centre' list. Those on the list are residential settings who have made application to gain approved status and they must satisfy stringent requirements including accounts for the last three years.

Let us assume that the woman is selling her house and wishes to enter a private home.

The owner of the home will have costed the fees per week necessary to provide the standard of care acceptable for registration. Staff salaries as well as household heating, lighting, repairs, and food have to be included.

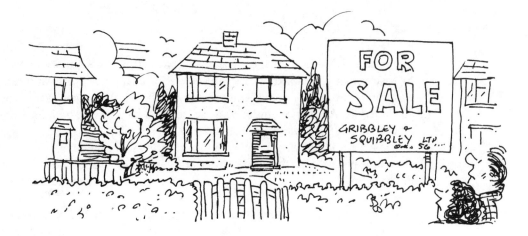

Proceeds from the sale of a house may be used to pay for residential care

If the woman accepts her place there, arrangements will be made to invest the proceeds from the sale of her house and regular payment will be made to the home. Any state or private pension she is entitled to will be hers in addition to the proceeds from the sale of her house. If there is ever a shortfall between the woman's assessed ability to pay the fees and the fees of the home, then it may be possible to have a 'top up' from the local authority in addition to her own payment. If there is no such facility then application could be made to charities or it might be possible to apply for a grant. In very rare cases the person has to move to a local authority home.

In the event that the woman has no property to sell then the local authority will pay the fees at a negotiated fixed rate in a private home or offer a place in a local authority home. The woman is still entitled to her state pension, but this is taken in part payment to the home with a percentage retained by the individual for personal expenses.

The late eighties and early nineties have seen a change of philosophy towards group living. Here efforts have been made to provide small units for perhaps eight people who have their own bedroom and share a sitting area and dining room. There may be several such small units within a much larger unit or home. The idea is to have a more personal approach which is aimed at supporting individuality. It is easy to feel isolated and lost in a very much larger group of forty, a feeling of being a number perhaps instead of an individual.

The National Health Service and Community Care Act 1990 gives the individual the right to choose the residential establishment they wish to take up residence in. The local authority has a duty to uphold that right wherever possible and to make the necessary arrangements. Empowering clients to make choices and ensuring that personal rights are maintained is now a key priority for all Health and Social Care settings.

Resources in terms of buildings and equipment are only a part of the equation in providing a caring environment. Staffing is an issue in terms of both the number of staff and the skills and knowledge they possess. It is people who make the difference between a caring environment or just a place to eat and sleep!

Care values

The values of caring are well expressed in the 'O' Unit of National Vocational Qualifications in the health and care field. This value base encompasses the duties and requirements of working in an anti-racist and anti-discriminatory way with clients of all ages and abilities.

Look again at the values described in detail in Chapter 1. Look too at the policies available in each care setting regarding codes of practice. You may wish to gain copies of the codes of practice recommended by the United Kingdom Central Council (UKCC) for Nurses, Health Visitors and Midwives, or British Association of Social Workers (BASW). Look too at the local authority community care plan and the Black Community Care Charter from the National Association of Race Equality Advisors.

Evidence opportunity

- Draw up a code of practice which you would advocate if you were the manager of a care organisation. You will need to identify the client group and justify your recommendations to ensure a high quality of life was available to all who use your organisation.
- Look at the Charter for Social Care and think of the small units in a residential setting. Living with a smaller group still has its problems as any member of a family group will appreciate. There will be times when there are differences of opinion, yet the chances of being able to express an opinion and to effect some control of one's life is arguably greater in a smaller unit than in a much larger one. What do you think? Analyse your thoughts and discuss them with others in the care field.

Culture of the environment

Other factors involved in the environment can best be considered by reference to the culture of the environment. The culture of the environment is the unwritten 'rules', 'the way things are done here'. This will depend on the staff team developing a clear philosophy regarding the kind of care they intend to offer. This will be influenced by the overall philosophy as described by the local authority, Health Service, voluntary organisation or private owner. The philosophy is often expressed as a mission statement which outlines the goals the provider intends to achieve in this particular service area.

Evidence opportunity

See if you can gain access to a variety of mission statements from different service providers and look at the similarities and note any differences.

Empowerment

Individuals should be empowered to take control of their own lives by being given choices and being encouraged to make decisions for themselves. Empowerment is a key element in the philosophy of care in Health and Social Care in the 1990s.

Empowerment means, for example, ensuring that information is shared so that an individual can make an informed decision about a course of action even if that involves taking a risk, for instance, taking control of administering their own medication. It is about respecting an individual's wishes regarding when they want to get up, go to bed or take a bath, etc. It is about access to personal files and the right to an advocate for those who feel they are unable to express themselves clearly.

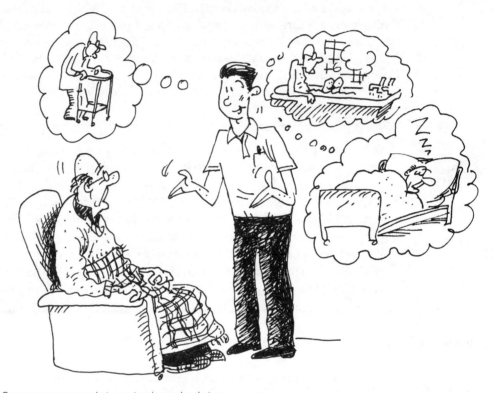

Empowerment means being assisted to make choices

All of this places the power with the individual and therefore reduces the power of the carer. People who have been working in the care field for some time may find this concept difficult to deal with at first. It challenges the ways that were accepted as good practice in the past and therefore questions the way individuals perceive themselves in their professional role – this may be seen as a threat to identity.

Instruments of change

What has brought about this change? Government legislation in the last decade has sought to ensure the health and well-being of people in care and in the community. This has resulted in regulations concerning:

- the registration of homes
- health and safety
- food hygiene and handling
- building regulations
- finance

- employment
- equal opportunities.

In turn the legislation reflects the concern of the general public in these areas so that provision is made to protect people in Britain through law. For example, the feminist movement in the late sixties and early seventies did much to bring about the Sex Discrimination Act 1975 in order to address the discrimination faced by women in employment. Equally the Race Relations Act 1976 aims to redress the imbalance and discrimination in employment of black people.

Pressure groups working for specific sections of the community aim to improve the quality of life for those who are their special interest; for example, Childline was set up in response to incidents of child abuse in some residential schools and children's homes. Age Concern works for elders and Mind works for people with mental ill-health.

Evidence opportunity

You may wish to focus on a particular pressure group and investigate the ways in which they work to raise public and government awareness of pertinent issues facing their client group. Prepare a presentation of your findings.

Staffing issues

Staff supervision and planned staff development is needed to explore any new philosophy. Staff supervision will assist staff to appreciate the basis for a particular concept, enabling them to re-evaluate their practice and grasp new concepts. In turn this may enable a carer to reaffirm their role and therefore their identity as a carer. Carers are still needed to provide a service but they now work to ensure that an individual is aware of their rights and encouraged to claim the right to live in dignity. Rights also include respect for individual differences in relation to religion, culture or sexuality. Respecting others may provide the satisfaction in the job that taking control and 'doing for others' had in the past.

Evidence opportunity

Choose two very different care organisations: one might be a private residential setting and another a community home for people moving from a longstay hospital. Another alternative might be a local authority residential setting or a residential setting run by a voluntary organisation.
- Look at the care environment provided by each setting. Take note of the resources in terms of the physical environment and staffing and note the ethos of each place.
- Try to identify any outside pressure group(s) which have been instrumental in ensuring improved quality of care.
- Examine the legislation which applies to the establishments and see how this is being met.
- Analyse and evaluate your findings and prepare a written case study of each to present to your study group for GNVQ.

There are many forms of caring environments providing care and support to people of all ages and abilities. The buildings may be large or small. They may be owned by the State, educational, health or voluntary organisations, or by private individuals.

This chapter has looked at the many factors, including legal and financial constraints, placed on staff working to provide a service to others in the health and care field. The final comment has to be that *you*, the carer, is the person responsible for ensuring that all for whom you care are offered a high quality service which meets their individual needs.

SECTION TWO – Summary

Advocate

To work with and to represent another person who is unable to negotiate their rights to services due to a learning or physical disability or for whom English is a second language.

Appraisal

A method to work with staff to identify their strengths within their work role. It is often used to identify staff development needs for the individual.

Assertion

The ability to state what you want, to express an opinion. To have the confidence to speak up for yourself without becoming aggressive or defensive.

Black person

Sociological term referring to anybody who is not white.

Business acumen

Having a flair for business.

Care manager

Someone who holds a budget for arranging the delivery of social care services in the community.

Community care

A legal term referring to service being provided for in the community. The concept is based on people having more power and say in what they want. Identified needs are met in discussion with professionals.

Competitive tendering

Applications are invited from outside the organisation to provide services.

Culture

The norms and values held by a particular group. This may be expressed through music, art, food, religion and behaviour.

Decentralisation

Where central or local government shift their power downwards towards operational staff, e.g. where large Town Halls allow small offices in the community to have their own budgets and make decisions locally.

Devolved budget

Senior managers handing over the operation and control of a budget to junior managers.

Dysfunctional group

A group unable to work together as a team often having many sub-groups, each with their own agenda.

Empathy

The ability to try and perceive the world from another person's point of view to gain a better understanding of them.

Empowerment

To give or delegate power. The process of making someone feel more powerful.

Functional group

A group able to work together having reached a stage where members accept the norms of the group thus enabling members to complete the task of the group.

Genuineness

Being sincere.

Group

More than three people who have a common cause for being together.

Group culture

The unwritten rules developed by a collection of people enabling them to establish acceptable behaviour by all members.

Group dynamics

A term used to describe the scientific study of groups. The term also applies to the processes of group activities.

Group norms

The commonly accepted attitudes and values held by a particular group to enable the group to function.

Interaction

The process of communication between the sender and receiver.

Individualism

Political term used by the Thatcher government which promoted the idea that people should make their own way in the world as individuals rather than rely on the State to help them.

Induction

A period of basic training to familiarise a new member of staff to the job.

Infrastructure

The basic structure of an organisation or system.

Leadership

Term given to leading or directing others. There are many styles of leadership and theories of how to use it.

Legislative duty

What the law directs you to do.

Legislative power

What the law enables you to do if you choose.

Management by objectives

Systems approach to planning. Linking your own planning to the needs of the organisation.

Mission statement

An organisation's overall aim.

Network

Interaction with a wide range of individuals from different establishments or disciplines to achieve an objective.

Norm

A sociological term to describe the basic pattern accepted by a given social group.

Opting out

A term when a publicly funded organisation takes up the government's offer to opt out of state control funding and manage its own budget.

Operational planning

The day to day planning of an organisation.

Organisation

Any group that is structured to work towards a goal.

Perception

Here it is used to mean the way an individual views and understands their world.

Performance related pay

Pay or bonus on achieving set targets.

Philanthropy

Giving one's time towards charitable works.

Prejudice

An opinion formed beforehand and which shows bias.

Private market

Organisations which offer caring services but operate on a profit basis.

Privatisation

Government process to change state owned and operated business into private operations.

Productivity

Yielding favourably. Producing a favourable amount.

Provider services

Services which are offered from organisations which only deliver and provide the service that is required.

Purchasing roles

The role someone plays in assessment or commissioning for services, e.g. care manager.

Purchasing services

Organisations which assess and commission other organisations to provide the service.

Quality assurance

A means of ensuring that standards are met by all people involved in the service.

Quality indicator

A yardstick to measure standards.

Reorganisation

When a local authority restructures, undergoing massive change.

Residential care

Accommodation which is provided for a person who is in need as defined by the National Assistance Act 1948.

Role ambiguity

Conflicting expectations of a given role in a particular situation. A new senior staff member unclear as to the boundaries of the role and the expectations of others.

Role conflict

Two very different demands made of an individual, e.g. for a doctor treating her own son for a serious injury the conflict is between the professional role and the maternal role.

Role model

A person to be looked up to and respected. Trying to be like that individual; e.g. many young people try to dress and act like a famous person. In the work setting it is modelling oneself on a member of staff deemed to be 'good at their job'.

Self-concept

The idea a person holds about themselves, i.e. how they perceive themselves.

Self-esteem

The value an individual places on themselves. Someone with low self-esteem will feel that they are of little value.

Siblings

Brothers and sisters of an individual.

Social role

The 'part' an individual plays in a given social setting, e.g. parent, carer.

Social status

The value placed on the role of an individual. This varies between cultures; e.g. in many Eastern cultures elders are deemed to have high social status as they have a wealth of knowledge and experience.

Socialisation

The process by which an individual learns acceptable behaviour within a particular group, i.e. the culture.

Staff appraisal

A system which employers operate to assess how well their staff are working.

Statutory care

Care which is provided by a legal order, e.g. Care Order for children.

Statutory guidance

Government guidance which follows legislation. It is not law but there are strong recommendations that organisations such as local authorities implement them.

Strategic planning

Long-term planning which an organisation invests in.

Sub-group

A group of people who form a smaller group within a larger group. This may be at the request of the members of the large group to achieve a particular aim. It may be that some people become disillusioned with the members/actions of the larger group and choose to break away; this could lead to group dysfunction.

Supervision

A system which an employer operates to support, train and develop its employees to ensure task completion.

Team

More than a purpose, a task. Working together effectively.

Trust status

The term often given to organisations which opt out of State control, e.g. hospitals.

Value

A belief held by an individual or a group of individuals, concerning the worth of an issue, e.g. valuing freedom of speech.

SECTION TWO – References and further reading

References

Adair, J., *Effective Team Building* (Pan, 1987)

Adair, J., *Effective Leadership* (Gower, 1989)

Ausubel, D.P. and Robinson, F.G., *School Learning* (Holt, Rinehart and Winston, 1969)

Bale, R.F., *Small Groups: Studies in Social Interaction* (Knopf, 1965)

Bartlett, F.C., *Remembering* (Cambridge University Press, 1932)

Benne, K.D. and Sheats, P., 'Functional Roles of Group Members' (1948) *Journal of Social Issues* **4**(2), 41–49

Douglas, T., *Groupwork Practice* (Tavistock Press, 1976)

Douglas, T., *A Handbook of Common Groupwork Problems* (Tavistock/Routledge, 1991)

Cattell, R.B. and Child, D., *Motivation and Dynamic Structure* (Holt, Rinehart and Winston, 1975)

Centre for Policy on Ageing, *Home Life* (Hare, 1984)

Glasser, R., *How to Get Extraordinary Performance from Ordinary People* (Organisation Design & Development Inc., 1987)

Handy, C., *Understanding Organisations* (Penguin, 1985)

Hare, A.P., *A Handbook of Small Group Research*, 2nd edn (Free Press, 1976)

Harvey-Jones, J., *The Age of Unreason* (Collins, 1989)

Harvey-Jones, J., *Making it Happen* (Fontana, 1990)

Hey, A., 'Organising teams, Alternative Patterns' in M. Marshall *et al.* (eds), *Team work for and against* (British Association of Social Work, Birmingham, 1979), pp. 25–36

Hull, C.L., *Principles of Behaviour* (Appleton-Century-Crofts, 1943)

Kelly, G.A., *A Theory of Personality – A Theory of Personal Constructs* (Norton, 1955)

Lewin, K., *Resolving Social Conflicts: Selected Papers on Group Dynamics* (Harper, 1948)

Marris, P., *Loss and Change* (Routledge, 1993)

Maslow, A.H., 'A Theory of Human Motivation' (1943) Psychol. Rev. 50

Oakley, A., *Sex Gender and Society* (Maurice Temple Smith, 1972)

Scott, T. and Payne, C., *Developing Supervision Teams In Field & Residential Social Work* Part I–II (NISW, 1982)

Scraggs, T. *et al.*, *Managing to Care* (Macmillan, 1993)

Sherif, M. and Sherif, C.W., *An Outline of Social Psychology* (Harper and Row, 1956)

Skinner, B.F., *Science and Human Behaviour* (Macmillan, 1953)

Thompson, N., *Anti-Discriminatory Practice* (Macmillan, 1993)

Tossell, D. and Webb, R., *Inside the Caring Services* (Hodder & Stoughton, 1988)

Tuckman, B.W., 'Developmental Sequences in Small Groups' (1965) *Psychological Bulletin* 63

Tuckman, B.W. and Jensen, M.A.C., 'Stages of Small Group Development Revisited' (1977) *Group and Organisational Studies* 2.

Wagner, G., *A Positive Choice* (HMSO, 1988)

Webb, A. and Hobdell, M., 'Co-ordination and Teamwork in the Health and Personal Social Services', Ch. 6 in S. Lonsdale, A. Webb and T. Briggs (eds), *Teamwork in the Personal Social Services and Health Care* (Manpower Monograph No. 14) (London P.S.S.C., 1980)

References on legislation regarding health and safety

The Food Hygiene (General) Regulations 1970 (S.I. 1970 No. 1172)
The main objective was to prevent food poisoning. Emphasis is placed on the prevention of contamination.

The Food Hygiene Act 1984
Relates to food to be consumed by humans in terms of storage, handling, preparation and premises. This applied to all food premises except Crown property, e.g. Health Authorities and their property.

The National Health Service (Amendment Act) 1986
Health Authorities and their properties lose Crown immunity for the purpose of food and health and safety legislation.

The Health and Safety at Work Act 1974
A completely new approach to health, safety and welfare for those in employment and the general public. Management must provide training to ensure high standards of health and safety are achieved. Employers must provide and implement a written health and safety policy and ensure that all staff are aware of it.

The Food Hygiene Act 1990
Minimum requirements laid down for the cleanliness and maintenance of food premises and equipment. This includes handling, preparation of food and details regarding the hygiene of food handlers.

The Food Hygiene (Amendment) Regulations 1990
Legal requirements for the temperature control of food. Prevention of contamination is the major focus. Details regarding the premises, equipment, washing and toilet facilities, i.e. there must be separate wash-basins for washing hands before the preparation of food.

Further suggested reading

Baugh, W.E., *Introduction to Social Services and Community Services*, 6th edn (Macmillan, 1992)

Braham, P. *et al.*, *Racism and Antiracism* (Open University, 1992)

Coulshed, V., *Management in Social Work* (Macmillan, 1992)

Egan, G., *The Skilled Helper*, 3rd edn (Brookes/Colle)

Moore, S., *Social Welfare Alive* (Stanley Thornes, 1993)

Murgatroyd, S. *Counselling and Helping* (British Psychological Society, 1988)

Nelson-Jones, R. *Human Relationship Skills* (Cassell, 1986)

Payne, P. *Working in Teams* (Macmillan, 1982)

Polras, S. *Systematic Problem Solving and Decision Making* (Kogan Page, 1989)

Tunnicliffe, H. *et al.*, *A-B-C of Community Care* (Pepar, 1993)

Index